Dreaming and Nightmares

Guest Editor

J.F. PAGEL, MS, MD

SLEEP MEDICINE CLINICS

www.sleep.theclinics.com

June 2010 • Volume 5 • Number 2

SAUNDERS an imprint of ELSEVIER, Inc.

W.B. SAUNDERS COMPANY
A Division of Elsevier Inc.

1600 John F. Kennedy Boulevard • Suite 1800 • Philadelphia, PA 19103-2899

http://www.sleep.theclinics.com

SLEEP MEDICINE CLINICS Volume 5, Number 2
June 2010, ISSN 1556-407X, ISBN-13: 978-1-4377-1872-0

Editor: Sarah E. Barth
Developmental Editor: Donald Mumford

Sleep Medicine Clinics (ISSN 1556-407X) is published quarterly by Elsevier Inc., 360 Park Avenue South, New York, NY 10010-1710. Months of issue are March, June, September and December. Business and Editorial Offices: 1600 John F. Kennedy Blvd., Ste. 1800, Philadelphia, PA 19103-2899. Customer Service Office: 3251 Riverport Lane, Maryland Heights, MO 63043. Periodicals postage paid at New York, NY and additional mailing offices. Subscription prices are $150.00 per year (US individuals), $76.00 (US residents), $346.00 (US institutions), $185.00 (foreign individuals), $106.00 (foreign residents), and $381.00 (foreign institutions). Foreign air speed delivery is included in all *Clinics* subscription prices. All prices are subject to change without notice. **POSTMASTER:** Send change of address to *Sleep Medicine Clinics*, Elsevier Health Sciences Division, Subscription Customer Service, 3251 Riverport Lane, Maryland Heights, MO 63043 Customer Service, (orders, claims, online, change of address): **Elsevier Health Sciences Division, Subscription Customer Service, 3251 Riverport Lane, Maryland Heights, MO 63043. Tel: 1-800-654-2452 (U.S. and Canada); 314-447-8871 (outside U.S. and Canada). Fax: 314-447-8029. E-mail: journals customerservice-usa@elsevier.com (for print support); journalsonlinesupport-usa@elsevier.com (for online support).**

Reprints. For copies of 100 or more of articles in this publication, please contact the Commercial Reprints Department, Elsevier Inc., 360 Park Avenue South, New York, NY 10010-1710. Tel.: 212-633-3812; Fax: 212-462-1935; E-mail: reprints@elsevier.com.

Printed and bound in the United Kingdom

Transferred to Digital Print 2011

GOAL STATEMENT

The goal of *Sleep Clinics of North America* is to keep practicing physicians up to date with current clinical practice by providing timely articles reviewing the state of the art in patient care.

ACCREDITATION

The *Sleep Clinics of North America* is planned and implemented in accordance with the Essential Areas and Policies of the Accreditation Council for Continuing Medical Education (ACCME) through the joint sponsorship of the University of Virginia School of Medicine and Elsevier. The University of Virginia School of Medicine is accredited by the ACCME to provide continuing medical education for physicians.

The University of Virginia School of Medicine designates this educational activity for a maximum of 15 *AMA PRA Category 1 Credits*™ for each issue, 60 credits per year. Physicians should only claim credit commensurate with the extent of their participation in the activity.

The American Medical Association has determined that physicians not licensed in the US who participate in this CME activity are eligible for a maximum of 15 *AMA PRA Category 1 Credits*™ for each issue, 60 credits per year.

Credit can be earned by reading the text material, taking the CME examination online at http://www.theclinics.com/home/cme, and completing the evaluation. After taking the test, you will be required to review any and all incorrect answers. Following completion of the test and evaluation, your credit will be awarded and you may print your certificate.

FACULTY DISCLOSURE/CONFLICT OF INTEREST

The University of Virginia School of Medicine, as an ACCME accredited provider, endorses and strives to comply with the Accreditation Council for Continuing Medical Education (ACCME) Standards of Commercial Support, Commonwealth of Virginia statutes, University of Virginia policies and procedures, and associated federal and private regulations and guidelines on the need for disclosure and monitoring of proprietary and financial interests that may affect the scientific integrity and balance of content delivered in continuing medical education activities under our auspices.

The University of Virginia School of Medicine requires that all CME activities accredited through this institution be developed independently and be scientifically rigorous, balanced and objective in the presentation/discussion of its content, theories and practices.

All authors/editors participating in an accredited CME activity are expected to disclose to the readers relevant financial relationships with commercial entities occurring within the past 12 months (such as grants or research support, employee, consultant, stock holder, member of speakers bureau, etc.). The University of Virginia School of Medicine will employ appropriate mechanisms to resolve potential conflicts of interest to maintain the standards of fair and balanced education to the reader. Questions about specific strategies can be directed to the Office of Continuing Medical Education, University of Virginia School of Medicine, Charlottesville, Virginia.

The faculty and staff of the University of Virginia Office of Continuing Medical Education have no financial affiliations to disclose.

The authors/editors listed below have identified no professional or financial affiliations for themselves or their spouse/partner:

Sarah Barth (Acquisitions Editor); Cynthia Brown, MD (Test Author); G. William Domhoff, PhD; Mylène Duval, PhD(c); Gary Fireman, PhD; Ernest Hartmann, MD; Milton Kramer, MD; Ross Levin, PhD; Tore Nielsen, PhD; J.F. Pagel, MS, MD (Guest Editor); Alan B. Siegel, PhD; Carlyle Smith, PhD; and Antonio Zadra, PhD.

The authors/editors listed below identified the following professional or financial affiliations for themselves or their spouse/partner:

Barry Krakow, MD owns and operates www.nightmaretreatment.com, www.sleeptreatment.com, and www.sleepdynamictherapy.com, markets and sells Insomnia Cures, Turning Nightmares into Dreams, and Sound Sleep, Sound Mind, owns and operates Maimonides Sleep Arts & Sciences, and is the president of the Sleep & Human Health Institute.
Teofilo Lee-Chiong Jr, MD (Consulting Editor) is on the Advisory Board/Committee for the American College of Chest Physicians and the American Academy of Sleep Medicine.
Michael Schredl, PhD is an industry funded research/investigator for Inc Research, Dusseldorf, Germany.
Lawrence Scrima, PhD, DABSM owns stock in Sepracor and Xenoport, and is an industry funded research/investigator for Pfizer.

Disclosure of Discussion of Non-FDA Approved Uses for Pharmaceutical Products and/or Medical Devices.

The University of Virginia School of Medicine, as an ACCME provider, requires that all faculty presenters identify and disclose any off-label uses for pharmaceutical and medical device products. The University of Virginia School of Medicine recommends that each physician fully review all the available data on new products or procedures prior to clinical use.

TO ENROLL

To enroll in the *Sleep Clinics of North America* Continuing Medical Education program, call customer service at 1-800-654-2452 or visit us online at www.theclinics.com/home/cme. The CME program is available to subscribers for an additional fee of $99.95.

Sleep Medicine Clinics

THE CLINICS ARE NOW AVAILABLE ONLINE!

Access your subscription at:
www.theclinics.com

Contributors

CONSULTING EDITOR

TEOFILO LEE-CHIONG Jr, MD
Professor of Medicine and Chief, Division
of Sleep Medicine, National Jewish Health;
Associate Professor of Medicine, University
of Colorado Denver School of Medicine,
Denver, Colorado

GUEST EDITOR

J.F. PAGEL, MS, MD
Associate Clinical Professor, Department of
Family Medicine, School of Medicine, University
of Colorado; Medical Director, Sleep Disorders
Center of Southern Colorado; Sleepworks Sleep
Laboratory, Colorado Springs, Colorado

AUTHORS

G. WILLIAM DOMHOFF, PhD
Distinguished Research Professor of Psychology,
University of California, Santa Cruz, Santa Cruz,
California

MYLÈNE DUVAL, PhD(c)
Clinical Psychologist, Surgery/Traumatology Unit,
Centre Hospitalier Universitaire Sainte Justine,
Montreal, Quebec, Canada

GARY FIREMAN, PhD
Professor and Chair, Department of Psychology,
Suffolk University, Boston, Massachusetts

ERNEST HARTMANN, MD
Professor of Psychiatry, Department
of Psychiatry, Tufts University School of Medicine,
Boston, Massachusetts; RFist Editor-in-Chief,
Dreaming

BARRY KRAKOW, MD
Medical Director, Maimonides Sleep Arts &
Sciences, Ltd., Maimonides International
Nightmare Treatment, Sleep & Human Health
Institute, Albuquerque, New Mexico

MILTON KRAMER, MD
Clinical Professor of Psychiatry, University
of Illinois, College of Medicine at Chicago,
Chicago, Illinois; Professor Emeritus in Psychiatry,
University of Cincinnati, Cincinnati, Ohio

ROSS LEVIN, PhD
Independent Practice, New York, New York

TORE NIELSEN, PhD
Professor, Department of Psychiatry, University
of Montreal; Director of Dream and Nightmare Lab,
Sacre-Coeur Hospital, Montreal, Quebec, Canada

J.F. PAGEL, MS, MD
Associate Clinical Professor, Department of
Family Medicine, School of Medicine, University
of Colorado; Medical Director, Sleep Disorders
Center of Southern Colorado; Sleepworks Sleep
Laboratory, Colorado Springs, Colorado

MICHAEL SCHREDL, PhD
Sleep Laboratory, Central Institute of Mental
Health, Mannheim, Germany

LAWRENCE SCRIMA, PhD, DABSM, FAASM
President and Director, Sleep-Alertness Disorders
Center-Consultants, Aurora, Colorado

ALAN B. SIEGEL, PhD
Assistant Clinical Professor, Department of
Psychology, University of California, Berkeley,
Berkeley, California

CARLYLE SMITH, PhD
Professor Emeritus of Psychology, Department
of Psychology, Trent University, Peterborough,
Ontario, Canada

ANTONIO ZADRA, PhD
Professor, Department of Psychology,
Université de Montréal, Montreal, Quebec,
Canada

Contents

reflect the ongoing memory consolidation process, but results do not support the idea that dreaming enhances this process.

Disturbed Dreaming and Emotion Dysregulation   229

Ross Levin, Gary Fireman, and Tore Nielsen

The AMPHAC/AND network is a vital component of the physiologic infrastructure of normal dreaming and likely influences the shaping of emotional imagery during normal and disturbed dreaming. By its endemic nature, dreaming is a naturally occurring self-regulatory process that may operate much like the emotional processing and habituation or desensitization that occurs during exposure therapy. Thus, the nature and quality of rapid eye movement sleep in particular likely interacts with these brain regions in the formation of dream imagery to facilitate the reduction or even elimination of fear-based memories in an ongoing attempt at achieving emotional homeostasis and optimize survival function.

The Dream Always Makes New Connections: The Dream is a Creation, Not a Replay   241

Ernest Hartmann

Every dream makes new connections, and every dream is a creative product, not a replay. This article summarizes evidence that even dreams usually thought of as replays—recurrent or repetitive dreams and post-traumatic stress disorder (PTSD) dreams—turn out to be new creations, rather than replays. This article discusses the implications of this view for the functions of dreaming and for the clinical use of dreams.

SECTION III: DISORDERED DREAMING AND NIGHTMARES

Frequency and Content of Dreams Associated with Trauma   249

Mylène Duval and Antonio Zadra

Sleep disturbances and dream-related disorders play a prominent role in trauma victims' clinical profile. Although some progress has been made in understanding the impact of sleep mechanisms and nightmares in the development, maintenance, and treatment of posttraumatic stress disorder (PTSD), little is known about the actual content of trauma-related dreams beyond the more strictly defined PTSD nightmares. This article presents key methodological issues, reviews findings on dream recall frequency following trauma exposure, examines the incidence of dream-related disorders as a function of trauma characteristics and personality variables, and reviews findings on the relationship between dream content and specific types of traumas. It is concluded that greater clinical and research efforts should be directed at understanding the natural course and impact of dream-related disorders as well as normal dream processes in trauma victims.

Dreaming Epiphenomena of Narcolepsy   261

Lawrence Scrima

This article examines the neuromechanisms and roles of dreaming in human emotions, motivation, and cognition through analysis of the sleep disorder narcolepsy, characterized by rapid eye movement sleep and related phenomena intrusion into working life, including intense dreaming. Methods of more productive and direct study of dreaming are suggested with narcolepsy patients, hypersomnolent patients, and normal subjects. Results from a few cogent studies with these populations are reviewed. The data surveyed support a theory of dreaming as a conduit between emotions, motivations, and higher cognitive processing, essential to memory consolidation, integration, personifying experiences, emotional stability, problem solving, and optimizing adaptive behavior.

Preface

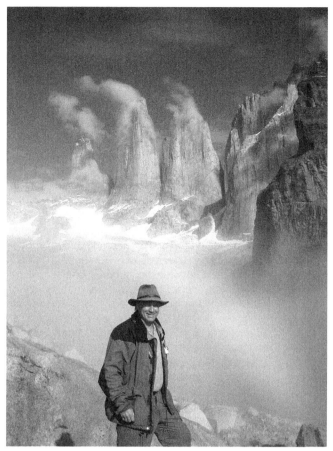

J.F. Pagel, MS, MD
Guest Editor

Dreaming is the longest studied yet least understood of cognitive states. The pedigree of dream study is ancient. The first decipherable human scripts inscribed into Mesopotamian clay 6,000 years ago include records of King Gudea's dreams that were perceived as messages from his gods. For the Ancient Greeks and Egyptians, it was most important to distinguish between "true dreams" (those that could be messages from god) and "false dreams." Rene Descartes built on this search for truth. He developed his scientific method while attempting to differentiate dreaming from external reality. The scientific study of dreams achieved prominence at the turn of the last century. Freud based his psychoanalytic theories of mental functioning on interpretations of dreams, focusing on the psychopathology associations of bizarre dreams and eventually giving us a definition of dreaming as "wish fulfillment." In the 1960s, the apparent realization that rapid eye movement (REM) sleep was dreaming broke through 500 years of belief in Cartesian dualism, leading us into a modern age of unitary activation-synthesis theory. If REM sleep is dreaming, philosophers and scientists should require no other evidence to conclude that mind—in neuroscientific actuality—equals brain.

In this new millennium, the scientific study of dreams has come full circle. Psychoanalysis, while useful as a cognitive model for the study of film, art, and intrapersonal psychodynamics, has generally failed as a treatment for psychiatric disease. After 50 years of dogma, most scientists and philosophers accept that research overwhelmingly

Sleep Med Clin 5 (2010) xi–xiii
doi:10.1016/j.jsmc.2010.01.012

sleep.theclinics.com

demonstrates that dreaming and REM sleep are doubly dissociable. REM sleep occurs without dreaming and dreaming without REM sleep.[1] Even the evidence supporting a special relationship between REM sleep and dreaming is equivocal, with only few a methodologically limited studies suggesting that REM sleep dream recall and content differs from the dreams of sleep onset.[2] Most sleep medicine physicians define dreaming as *mentation reported as occurring in sleep*. However, this definition contradicts the psychoanalytic definition for dream, by restricting dreaming to sleep irrespective of content. This definition also differs from the REM sleep–equals–dreaming model in requiring a dream report.

This perspective—that a dream report is required if REM sleep equals dreaming—is not universally accepted. With the advent of micropipette brain slice techniques, knock-out mice, and central nervous system scanning with functional magnetic resonance imaging, squib, and positron emission technology, we now understand far more about the REM sleep state than we understand about dreaming.[3] If REM sleep does not equal dreaming, the requirement for a dream report restricts scientific studies of dreaming to subjects capable of cognitive interaction (generally humans). Scientists loath to giving up the role of dreaming as a behavioral aspect of the REM sleep neurocognitive model have stretched the definition of dreaming to include parasomnias and the REM sleep–associated states of narcolepsy, with dreaming defined as any bizarre, hallucinatory mental activity occurring during sleep or while awake.[4,5] Theorists suggest that such mentation indicates the occurrence of REM sleep, whether occurring in polysomnographic REM sleep, in non-REM sleep, or even in waking.[6] The other sleep mentation is classified as non-REM sleep or sleep "mental activity" (See the article by Lawrence Scrima elsewhere in this issue for further exploration of this topic.). This approach preserves the REM sleep–equals–dreaming correlate, but requires a redefinition of both sleep states and dreaming.[7] Based on this perspective, the most commonly reported dreams, continuity dreams reflecting the experience of waking life, are not dreams.

Perhaps this is dreams' darkest hour. The percentage of scientific articles addressing dreaming peaked with the discovery of REMS but has now declined to the lowest level in 60 years (see the graph). What we know today about dreaming is far less than what we thought we knew a generation ago. Much older work is methodologically limited by lack of definition, small sample size, and constraints of theoretical perspective. Even among this issue's small sample

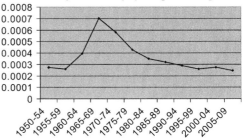

Papers on Dreaming - % of total published papers [Pubmed]

of dream scientists, definitions of dreaming vary so that different authors are writing about mutually exclusive topics—all called dreaming. It remains unclear, as well, as to what part, if any, of the highly developed REM sleep neurocognitive model applies to cognitive state of dreaming.

This issue provides a purview of the current approaches being used by major researchers involved in the scientific and clinical study of dreaming. Milton Kramer reviews the status of scientific rigor in dream research. Mark Schredl reviews our current understanding of variables affecting dream recall. Bill Domhoff reviews our current understanding of dream content, highlighting the lack of evidence that REM sleep dreaming differs in content from the dreaming associated with other sleep stages. Carlyle Smith addresses the association of REM sleep with learning and memory and the proposed role for dreaming in this process. My own article is an evidence-based review of the neurochemistry affecting dreaming and nightmares, indicating that the medications affecting dreaming differ from those affecting REM sleep. For those readers interested in maintaining their belief in dreaming as a REM sleep epiphenomenon, Lawrence Scrima suggests that narcolepsy may be an the ideal model for the study of dreaming.

This issue's clinical focus is reflected in its emphasis on the theory, diagnosis, and treatment of the most common of the parasomnias—nightmares. Ernest Hartmann highlights the contextual imagery involved in such powerful dreams. Mylène Duval and Antonio Zadra address our current understanding of nightmares, and Ross Levin addresses the apparent functions for nightmares in emotional processing. Barry Krakow and Antonio Zadra focus on treatment of the nightmares associated with post-traumatic stress disorder, while Alan Seigel addresses the current use of dream reports in clinical psychotherapy.

Many other and larger publications about dreams focus on phenomenology and theory.

This issue differs from those in its emphasis on scientific evidence, providing for the reader the best available review of the current status of dream science, as well as a review and assessment of clinical approaches to dreaming and nightmares. However, this issue has a prominent subtext that can be read in both its brevity and lack of positive conclusions: What we scientifically understand about both dreams and nightmares is profoundly limited. After 6000 years of study, this cognitive state remains both an enigma and an opening for the enterprising open-minded scientist fascinated by the unknown.

J.F. Pagel, MS, MD
Department of Family Medicine
School of Medicine
University of Colorado, CO, USA

Sleep Disorders Center of Southern Colorado
1619 North Greenwood, Suite 107, CO 81003, USA

Sleepworks Sleep Laboratory, Colorado Springs
1330 Quail Lake Loop, CO 80906, USA

E-mail address:
Pueo34@juno.com

REFERENCES

1. Solms M. Dreaming and REM sleep are controlled by different brain mechanisms. In: Pace-Schott E, Solms M, Blagtove M, et al, editors. Sleep and dreaming: scientific advances and reconsiderations. Cambridge (UK): Cambridge University Press; 2003. p. 51–8.

2. Domhoff GW. The scientific study of dreams; neural networks, cognitive development and content analysis. Washington, DC: American Psychological Association; 2003.

3. Pace-Schott EF. Postscript: recent findings on the neurobiology of sleep and dreaming. In: Pace-Schott EF, Solms M, Blagrove M, et al, editors. Sleep and dreaming: scientific advances and reconsiderations. Cambridge: Cambridge University Press; 2003. p. 335–50.

4. Pagel JF, Blagrove M, Levin R, et al. Defining dreaming—a paradigm for comparing disciplinary specific definitions of dream. Dreaming 2001;11(4): 195–202.

5. Pagel JF, Scrima L. Psychoanalysis and narcolepsy. In: Goswami M, Pandi-Perumal, Thorpy M, editors. Narcolepsy. Humana/Springer, in press.

6. Neilsen T. A review of mentation in REM and NREM sleep: "covert" REM sleep as a possible reconciliation of two opposing models. In: Pace-Schott E, Solms M, Blagtove M, et al, editors. Sleep and dreaming: scientific advances and reconsiderations. Cambridge (UK): Cambridge University Press; 2003. p. 59–74.

7. Pagel JF. The limits of dream—a scientific exploration of the mind/brain interface. Oxford (UK): Academic Press (Elsevier); 2008.

The Assessment of Dream Content: Methodological Considerations

Milton Kramer, MD[a,b,c],*

KEYWORDS

• Dreams • Collection • Quantification

DEFINITION

While discussing the study of dreams, it is essential to be clear on what does and what does not constitute a dream.[1] This is true for whatever one studies; the object of study must be delineated, or confusion and contradiction will be the inevitable consequence. This question was raised by the author in the symposium entitled "Dreams, dream content and their psychophysiologic correlates" at the First International Congress of the Association for the Psycho-physiological Study of Sleep in 1972.[2] The importance of the definition of the term dream was rejected in the discussion but recognized by the chair as a recurrent theme that remained unresolved. More recently, under the direction of the editor of this issue, James Pagel, MD, an effort has been undertaken to provide a definition for dream,[3] but it resulted in the conclusion that there was no single definition possible. After reviewing about 20 definitions of dreaming, it was concluded that definitions of dreaming have 3 characteristics: (1) an association with wake/sleep states, (2) recall, and (3) content.

It is not apparent what is meant when one says one is studying the dream. There is little agreement on what is encompassed and what is excluded in the concept "the dream." Nagera[4] provides Freud's most concise definition of the dream: "a dream is the (disguised) fulfillment of a (repressed) wish." The *American Heritage Dictionary of the English Language* says that the dream is "a series of images, ideas, and emotions occurring in certain stages of sleep."[5] Klinger[6] suggests that dreaming is (best) defined as any reportable mental event that occurs during periods of sleep. Malcolm,[7] a philosopher of mind, has stated that dreaming has the dream report as its criterion. Erickson[8] says, "A dream is the verbal report of a series of remembered images, mostly visual, which are usually endowed with affect." It is not possible, even with awakenings at night, to isolate the dream experience per se, and at best, one can only obtain a description of the experience. The most operational definition of the dream is that offered by Klinger, Malcolm, and Erickson, namely that the dream we study is really the dream report.

The process of defining is really not self evident. To define is to offer a precise meaning. Defining includes a description of the nature and basic qualities of the matter to be defined. Definition would require a delineation of the outline and form of the object of interest. The process of definition recognizes in what manner the object of definition is different from other similar things with which it may be confused and from which it needs to be distinguished. Applying these standards of definition to define the dream would require that the content, form, and limits of the dream be described in comparison to other things

[a] Department of Psychiatry, University of Illinois, College of Medicine at Chicago, 912 South Wood Street, Chicago, IL 60612, USA
[b] Department of Psychiatry, University of Cincinnati, 231 Bethesda Avenue, Cincinnati, OH 45267, USA
[c] 1110 North Lake Shore Drive, Apartment 23S, Chicago, IL, 60611, USA
* 1110 North Lake Shore Drive, Apartment 23S, Chicago, IL, 60611.
E-mail address: milton1929@yahoo.com

Sleep Med Clin 5 (2010) 183–191
doi:10.1016/j.jsmc.2010.01.005

with which it may be confused and from which it should be differentiated. Taub and colleagues[9] compared what the subjects described as a nightmare with a nightmare and a dream that they had experienced and found that the confabulated nightmare report was shorter in length and had more aggression, movement, intensity, and misfortune and was reported in a more organized manner than the nightmare they had experienced. The experienced nightmare and dream were of the same length, but the nightmare was more active and aggressive and had more misfortunes, color, and institutions. The dream must be captured (recalled, collected, and recorded), measured (quantified), and compared (appropriately).[10,11]

It is of special importance to be concerned about the methodological issues involved in studies of dreaming. The most fundamental problem is that the dream report is a report of a subjective experience for which there is no external (objective) marker. There has been serious concern that subjective events cannot be explored scientifically. Dennett[12] has pointed out quite convincingly that once first-person experiences are reported, they can be seen as texts and can be effectively examined using third-person techniques that are the hallmark of scientific undertakings.

PRE–RAPID EYE MOVEMENT STUDIES

In 1953, Ramsey[13] reviewed the pre–*rapid eye movement* (REM) scientific literature on dreams and provided the background for a review of the methodological issues in studying the dream. He restricted his review "to the more empiric and systematic studies of dreaming, particularly those in which some quantitative findings are reported." He included studies "if the results presented could be checked by repetition of the investigation." Because the studies were so poorly reported, he "adopted the policy of presenting findings whenever they were based on quantitative data even though an adequate basis for their evaluation was not included in the report." Ramsey cited 121 articles and books, 20 of which deal with 6 psychiatric entities. He concluded his review of the dream literature with a highly unfavorable evaluation of the quality of the research. He noted that only a few of the studies were so designed and reported that they could be repeated to confirm their findings. The dream studies were particularly weak in describing the population under study; for example, information on the sex, age, intelligence, health, economic status, and education of the subjects was rarely provided. The studies were too often based on limited or selected groups of subjects. Appropriate control groups were not used when comparative statements were made. Ramsey urged that more precise definitions be used in selecting and classifying various characteristics of dreams. He was of the opinion that statistical controls and treatment of the data was necessary, and as dream collection was based on interviewing the dreamer, controls for interviewing bias should be used.

DREAM RECALL
History

The factors that influence the recall of dreams must be understood and taken into account in any study of dreams. Freud[14] addressed this question and opined that the summary of the recall problem by Strumpell in 1871 was quite thorough. Strumpell recognized that forces that generally control recall in waking life would also operate to influence the recall of dreams. He recognized 8 such factors: (1) the intensity of the dream experience, which included its vividness and its dramatic intensity; (2) whether it was a single or repeated event, clearly the latter being more likely to be recalled but less likely to occur; (3) the disconnected and disorderly nature of the dream experience when organized as stories with meaning are easier to recall; (4) the distraction that waking provides leads to a fading of the dream experience[15]; (5) interest in dreaming may lead to an increase in recall (however, we found that those who expressed an interest in dreams actually had a lower recall of dreams)[16]; (6) state dependency, with dreaming occurring during one state, sleep, being recalled in another state, wakefulness, may well influence recall as Overton[17] has suggested; (7) dreams that may not be recalled on awakening may be recalled later when primed by some related waking thought; and (8) recalling a fragment may lead to filling the dream out with confabulated material to make it more organized, a sort of secondary revision that Freud described as occurring. Freud's contribution was to add repression to the factors that influence dream recall.

Experimental Studies of Factors in Dream Recall

What is the rate of dream recall? College students estimate that on average they have 2 to 3 dreams a week; 15% of these students report never recalling a dream and 5% report having more than 1 dream a night.[18] In an interview study of a statistically representative group of adults in the city of Cincinnati,[19] 61% were able to report a recent dream; gender and age were factors, with women (65%) more likely to report a dream than men(53%) and older subjects having lower recall rates than younger subjects.[20] Across 16 studies,[21] an awakening from REM sleep was likely to result in a dream report from 60% to 89% of the time, with a median of 74%. Individuals were able to recall 3 to 5 dreams from REM sleep awakenings but report only 1 dream every other day when in psychoanalytic treatment.[22]

What accounts for the selection process from 3 to 5 dreams a night to 1 every other day? We compared the dreams of 2 patients, one man and one woman, who reported at night to the technician and to the psychiatrist the next day or a day later.[23] The male subject reported 34 dreams from 46 REM period awakenings (74%), and the female subject had 54 reports from 60 awakenings (90%). The male subject reported 7 of the 34 plus 3 additional ones in the morning. The female subject reported 41 of the dream reports in the morning plus 7 that she didn't report at night. For both, major changes or deletions were 3 times more common than complete forgetting. The male subject reported to the psychiatrist only dreams that demonstrated his manliness and left out those with homosexual implications. The female subject often failed to tell the psychiatrist dreams that had thinly disguised critical or sexual themes. The most striking feature was that the 15 dream reports that were not told to the psychiatrist were those that expressed fears of psychiatry. The fidelity with which dreams were reported, the fact that the omitted dreams were as likely to be from the first half of the night as the second, and the fact that the number of dreams told the morning after or 24 hours later were essentially the same suggested that simple forgetting did not account for which dreams were being selected to be reported and that the interpersonal situation might be a determinant in the selection process.

A series of studies examining the effects of several factors that might influence the recall of dreams was conducted. It was found that varying the gender match of subject and experimenter[24] led to a 6% to 7% higher recall with the male experimenter. There were clear content differences such as more groups in dreams when the subject-experimenter pair was heterosexual. Cartwright and Kasniak[25] found that after watching an explicit heterosexual film, there was a 14% decrease in dream recall in a heterosexual group, whereas a homosexual group had only a 2.5% decrease. If adaptation to the laboratory took place, the likelihood of dreams being responsive to the interpersonal situation would be decreased. In subjects who slept for 20 consecutive nights in the laboratory and were awakened from each REM period,[26] there was no significant decrease

in dream recall. The effect of personality dimensions on dream recall was also studied.[27] REM dream reports for 3 nights and a 2-week dream diary were collected from 24 college students. Measures of anxiety, repression ego strength, and field independence were also obtained. There was no relationship between these personality variables and dream recall. We looked at the formal aspects of recall in schizophrenic patients,[28] as these factors had been found to be determiners of dream recall in normal people. The position and the number of dreams in the night significantly influenced its recall in the morning as we found a recency, a primacy, and an interference effect. Dramatically intense and longer dreams were also more likely to be reported. We compared the content of the dreams collected at night on 12 scales with those reported in the morning and found that groups were higher in the night dreams and individuals in the morning dreams. In a group of 22 normal subjects[29] who slept for 20 nights, content differences were found based on position of the dream in the night. We looked at the recall of dreams across the REM period and found increases in recall the further into the REM period the awakening occurs.[30] However, despite our studies that dream content is psychodynamically sensitive and that there are dream content differences based on the position of the dream in the night, it is the formal characteristics of recall that have to be given greater weight in accounting for what dream reported at night is recalled in the morning.

It has been observed that remembering dreams once awake is a difficult task. The difficulty may be related to what Overton[17] has described as state-dependent recall; events experienced in one state, sleep, are difficult to recall in another state, wakefulness. The connectedness of thematic content when awake is more alike and better before and after sleep than during the intervening dreams,[31] and these organizational differences suggest 2 different states of consciousness.

There are other factors that may influence dream recall, such as whether one has an interest in dreams or whether one is a good or poor sleeper. Comparison of 2-week sleep diaries of those who had an interest in dreams with those who did not showed that those with an interest in dreams reported fewer, not more, dreams.[16] Comparison of 2-week dream diaries of poor sleepers with those of good sleepers found that the poor sleepers reported more dreams.[32] Interference or distraction interferes with the recall of dreams.[15,28] Goodenough and colleagues[33] have shown that abrupt arousal from sleep increases the likelihood of a dream recall probably as it keeps the focus of the dreamer from shifting to waking issues. Disorganization of a dream report does not affect recallability, but the dreams of poor recallers are harder for others to remember than those of good recallers.[34] Repeated events are easier to recall, but dreams are usually singular events. The nightmare sufferer may have similar repeated dreams, but has a mental content much like people without nightmares and is only an average dream recaller.[35] The patient with *posttraumatic stress disorder* has only 50% of his dreams related to trauma but seems to select these trauma-related dreams for recall because they are more dramatic.[36] Dementia and age negatively effect dream recall.[37] Dream recall from non-REM awakenings ranges from 7% to 75%, depending on the standard for rating a report as a dream and the non-REM stage from which the subject was awakened, time since the last eye movements, the time of night of the awakening, and the expectations of the experimenters in regard to the possibility of recovering mental content.[38] Learning after awakening from stage 4 sleep was poorer than after awakening from stage 2 sleep, but after being awake for 8 minutes, the prior stage of sleep makes no difference in learning.[39] A carryover effect exists for awakenings from REM sleep as well.[40]

Several factors influence dream recall. The formal aspects of recall, particularly dream length and dramatic intensity, are of primary importance, with content-related factors being secondary. Intrinsic properties of the dream experience, that is, the length of time into REM, the time of night of the dream collection and the state of the brain, and prior stage of sleep or brain damage will also effect recall. Demographic factors and processes of rehearsal, consolidation, and level of arousal play a role as well.

An Arousal-Retrieval Theory of Dream Recall

Goodenough[41] divides dream forgetting into content-centered or memory-process–centered theories. Goodenough and Koulack[42] offer a hypothesis to account for the recall of dreams. They assume that a cognitive processing of the dream in short-term memory occurs in preparation for transfer to long-term memory. If the subject is insufficiently aroused, the cognitive process of coding, reorganizing, and labeling of memory is inadequate and transfer to long-term memory is impaired or does not occur. In addition, retrieval of the memory, if it is transferred, is more difficult or impossible. Distractions on awakening would interfere with the cognitive processing and transfer to long-term memory. As it is difficult to

recall any experience that occurs during sleep, content-based recall theories are less likely than memory-based theories to account for recall.

DREAM COLLECTION AND QUANTIFICATION
Introduction

We have on several occasions[1,10,11] reviewed issues related to the collection and measurement of the dream report. Several studies that bear on factors that effect the collection of dream reports have been enumerated in an earlier section. An essentially visual experience experienced in one state, sleep, which has to be reported verbally in another state, wakefulness, presents challenging problems. A brief review of my previous observations on dream collection will suffice for the present purposes.

Dream Report Collection

There are several collection factors that influence the content of the verbal dream report, and they include (1) the place in which the dream is experienced and reported, (2) the method of awakening the dreamer, (3) the context of the interpersonal situation in which the report is given, (4) the style of the collection interview, (5) the time of night and the stage of sleep from which the sleeper is awakened, (6) the method of recording the dream report, and (7) the type of subject from whom the dream is collected.

1. Dream reports collected in *different settings* have clear content differences. Sleeping at home or in the laboratory yields differences in dream content. Dreams collected in the laboratory are less intense and less vivid than those collected at home. When the circumstances are equated, no differences were found, although home dreams were more aggressive. The laboratory situation continues to be represented in dream reports for 3 weeks, with no adaptation occurring.
2. The *method of awakening* the subject, fast or slow, alters the frequency of recall. The faster the awakening the lesser the distraction and a recall is more likely. The nature of the awakening stimulus makes a difference, whether it is auditory, visual, or tactile. Dream incorporation is more easily accomplished with a verbal stimulus.
3. The real or imagined *interpersonal situation* in which the dream report is collected will influence what is reported and what is withheld. Factors such as familiarity between the dreamer and dream collector as well as the sex and status of the collector in relation to

the dreamer influences what will be reported and to whom. The relationship may be a changing one with time. Varying the dream collector has the potential to alter what is reported.

4. The *method and technique of the collection interview* can alter the dream report. Asking, "What were you dreaming?" may get a different response from "What was going through your mind before I awakened you?" Given the subtleties of the relationship and the demand characteristics of the situation, safeguards are necessary to prevent the interviewer obtaining what he wants to find.

5. The *time of night and stage of sleep* at which the dreamer is awakened will influence the probability, quantity, and quality of the recall. Content differences have been found between early and late, short and long, and interrupted and uninterrupted REM periods. What is recovered depends on how far into the REM period the awakening occurs.

6. The *method of recording* the dream will inevitably influence the report obtained. Verbal reports lead to longer and poorly organized reports, whereas writing leads to better-organized and shorter reports. The former is limited by the verbal facility of the dreamer and the latter by their written facility.

7. The *subject variables* have been shown to influence the probability of recall, that is, recallers versus nonrecallers, volunteers versus nonvolunteers, poor sleepers versus good sleepers. Male and female subjects have different fantasies about sleeping in the sleep laboratory. Men have concerns about being exploited and women about being raped.

Winget and Kramer[10] provide a detailed protocol for dream collection and measurement, which may prove helpful to investigators.

Measurement of Dream Reports

The core of scientific enterprises is to be able to reliably and validly quantitatively examine the object being studied. Quantification is essential in studying dreaming but unfortunately has been neglected. It has been readily assumed that the essential nature of the dream will be lost if it is treated quantitatively. In addition to the conviction that there is an ineffable aspect to the dream, which lends an appealing mystical quality to the dream, the psychoanalytic view that studying the manifest content, distracted from the search for the disguised latent dream thoughts, from the meaning of the dream, had discouraged efforts to measure the dream report systematically.

The verbal dream report usually becomes the text for measurement in psychological dream studies. There are several issues that need to be clear in undertaking measuring aspects of the dream report and they include (1) the verbal nature of the dream report, (2) the definition of the scoreable dream report text, (3) the effect of dream report length on the type of measurement to be made, (4) the methods of quantifying dream content, and (5) the reliability and validity of the measurement.[11]

1. The *verbal nature* of the dream report. The nature of the report raises 2 important issues. The first is that the report is so influenced by the verbal fluency of the subject that any content differences found within and between subjects may be alternatively explained on differences between the fluency of the subjects. There has been very limited study of subjects' describing an event and describing a dream. In a population study, we had subjects report a dream and an early memory and both had the same average length of 22 words. The need is for a similar laboratory study that compares subjects' length of words while awake and describing their dreams and some other experience that is of similar time length. Limitations in the case of the Hall-Van de Castle norms are that they are written and are not verbal and are of educated young adults and include only dream reports of 100 words or more. The writing out of dreams presents its own special concerns related to the writing skills of the subject and the difficulty in writing in a disorganized manner. The second issue is whether the content or form of the verbal report is different from other narrative fantasy productions such as thematic apperception test stories, verbal samples, or descriptions of early memories. A comparison of nonlaboratory dream reports with psychological tests in 28 studies showed inconsistent results. Comparing a patient's history to laboratory dreams and to psychological testing using a q-sort technique found significant relationships among the various data sources. The dream reported at night was more fragmentary than the same dream reported the next morning; a sort of secondary revision was occurring. The pre- and postsleep verbal samples were more related to each other, although further apart in time than the intervening dreams. The assumed uniqueness of the dream remains to be demonstrated.

2. *The text to be measured.* The verbal dream report text that is measured is some distilled

version of what was reported. The repetitions, contrasts with real life, exclusionary comments, associational remarks, and gratuitous comments and explanations are generally removed. The final dream text depends very much on the assumptions made about the dream experience. All of the report would be the basis for a possible psychoanalytic interpretation. Including the associations to a dream reported in therapy increases the presence of an affect from 58% to 96%. The results of a study may be altered by the assumptions about the dream text and are theoretically important, as many believe that the driving force for the dream is its affect.

3. *The length of the dream report.* The length of the report will effect what is found; generally, the longer the report the more items will be found. Simply dividing by length assumes a fixed relationship of word length to all items of potential interest, which does not seem to be the case. Other solutions that have been offered include limiting the study to dreams of a minimal length or to report scoreable items in terms of another item as a ratio. Using word length minimums excludes much of dream reporting; our population study had a mean length of 22 words. Freud published analyses of a 1-word, a 48-word and a 369-word dream. The use of ratios depends on the items chosen for study and that the dream is long enough for both items to appear. It might work if one is comparing in men and women the relationship of friendly to aggressive interactions but not if one looks at the relationship of physical activities to sadness in the psychotically depressed.

The process of quantifying the content of dream reports presents some major technical issues.[10] A usable measuring scheme should (1) state the assumptions in regard to the item or concept to be measured, (2) give well defined anchoring points, (3) list inclusive and exclusive examples for each scale point, (4) indicate the unit to be coded, (5) specify the contextual unit to be used in making scoring decisions, and (6) provide a scoring unit for deriving a total score. The other major technical question is how to deal with the intensity dimension. Nominal or category scales simply sort the content of the dream into various categories of items. An intensity dimension can be approximated by reporting the change in the number of items in a class. A dream with 6 people is more "peopled" than a dream with 2 people. If one undertakes to do an equal interval scale, where the distance between scale points is equal, one runs the risk of certain absurdities. If it is a

4-point heterosexual scale that has a heterosexual pair as point 1 and intercourse as point 4 then one has the absurdity of 4 instances of heterosexual pairs equaling 1 instance of intercourse.

4. *The reliability of measurement.* The reproducibility of measurement is essential to having any confidence in the measurement efforts. Ratings may be intra- or interjudge depending on the nature of the study and the number of judges that are being used. The assumption that the ratings will be stable once a rater is trained to an acceptable level of reliability denies the inevitable drift that occurs in human judgment. Reliability is inflated if absence of the item in question is common. Reliability, accuracy of measurement, sets the upper limit for validity.

5. *The validity of measurement.* The validity of the dream content scoring is established as validity would be in any other psychological circumstance. The scoring system should have face or content validity, that is, the scale content should be appropriate to the concept being measured. The scale should show construct validity, that is, the scale should be measuring the correct concept, the scale items should be related to each other, and the scale should do what is was intended to do, for example, angry people should have higher anger scores. Lastly and perhaps most importantly, the scales should have criterion or predictive validity, that is, the scales should predict consequences or outcomes. The Hall-Van de Castle character scale demonstrates face validity in the extent to which types of characters can be scored; has construct validity in that it delineates types of people (therefore categorization by gender; age; familiarity; and occupational, social, and family roles); has construct validity, as applying it has shown that character types are understandably related to psychiatric diagnosis, that is, the stranger to schizophrenics and family character roles to psychotically depressed patients.

Conclusion

The quantification of the ineffable dream report is possible from several different aspects without trivializing the dream's essence. The measurement of the dream report can serve to solidify clinical observations by separating reproducible from nonreproducible results, and given the large number of scaling systems, need not lead to the endless proliferation of dream measurement systems, as combining scales can often capture the concept of interest. The dream report is both variable and stable across short and long periods, reflecting the state and trait characteristics of the dreamer. The examination of quantified manifest dream content can lead to meaningful insights about the so-called deeper meanings of the dream experience.

THE APPLICATION OF METHODOLOGICAL RIGOR IN DREAM CONTENT STUDIES
Introduction

It is appropriate to examine the dream literature to see if adequate attention has been paid to methodological issues since the resurgence of interest in the dream after the discovery of REM sleep and the methodological critique of the pre-REM dream literature by Ramsey[13]. We have undertaken a survey of the entire periodic literature from 1958 to 1975[43] and updated it in a survey covering the years to 2005.[44] Combined we obtained 1906 titles and chose to focus on a subset of the literature dealing with the dreams of psychiatric patients with major illnesses, about 169 studies. We categorized the studies along 53 parameters that covered the areas of (1) the type, nature, and site of the studies; (2) the adequacy of the description of the patient sample; (3) the adequacy of the description of the control sample; (4) the method of dream content collection; (5) the method of scoring dream content; (6) the nature of the statistical analyses; (7) the dream content results obtained. The reviews established only the presence or absence of the various categories and not their adequacy, with the exception of the statistical categorization.

The Type, Nature, and Site of Studies

Two-thirds to three-quarters of the dream reports were studies and not case reports. Unfortunately, they have become increasingly descriptive and are less often separate group studies, that is, comparing 2 groups. Three-quarters are nonlaboratory in nature, so the complete range of the dreamers' experience is not being captured. The control group in the separate group studies is three-quarters of the time another sick group, so illness is controlled.

The Adequacy of the Description of the Patient Group

The sample size was and remained acceptable. The basis for the diagnosis was given only half the time, and treatment, physical, or pharmacologic information was given a quarter to a third of the time. Demographic variables of sex and race were provided almost universally, whereas race, education, marital status, and social class only a quarter of the time or less. Health was mentioned in more recent studies a third of the time, and most studies had gone from being done on hospital patients to being done on outpatients.

The Adequacy of Description of the Control Sample

The percentage of separate group studies was small and those done in the laboratory was even smaller, but the number of subjects was acceptable. The reporting of the basis for establishing the selection and diagnosis of patients in the control group and whether they were being treated had improved considerably from 1975 to 2005. The inclusion of demographic variables mimicked what was found for the patient group. The same was true for the health and site of residence of the control group. The overall reporting of significant subject variables was better in the separate group studies than in the descriptive studies.

The Method of Dream Content Collection

The reporting of the number of nights or days of study, the number and percentage of dreams collected, by who and when they were collected, the mode of awakening and recording the report, and the protocol for obtaining the report and associations were generally specified in 50% to 60% of studies and decreased between the time of the 2 reviews. Any conviction in regard to describing fully the dream collection process not only had not improved but also had apparently weakened.

The Method of Scoring Dream Content

This category of methodology is most remarkable in how little attention is paid to it in the dream studies. Protocol preparation, "blind" raters, and reliability of scoring are described in less than 20% of studies. The number of raters and type and source of the rating instrument are not given 60% of the time. If one cannot assess how and what was measured, no credence can be given to any study result.

The Nature of the Statistical Analyses

Statistical results have been reported in 33% to 41% of the studies, declining from 1975 to 2005. The tests are appropriate to the design and data and had significant results in 70% to 81% of cases. The low number of studies that reported a statistical analysis of their data reduces much of the dream literature to anecdotes.

The Dream Content Results Obtained

The methodological limitations of the dream literature devoted to the dreams of psychiatric patients makes it very difficult to accept the results of these studies. If we add the standard of independent replicability, we reduce considerably our knowledge of the dream life of psychiatric patients and the contribution that studying the dreams of psychiatric patients could make to understanding their illness. For example, the literature has suggestions that the dreams of schizophrenics are unrealistic; affectively neutral; openly hostile, with the hostility being directed at the dreamer; less blatantly sexual than the dreamer's waking life, with the dream action focused on the dreamer who finds himself most often with strangers. We would limit our description using a verifiability standard to their dreams being more hostile, more affective, with more strangers, and having more evidence of the schizophrenic thought disorder than nonschizophrenics.

Conclusion

It is apparent that the literature on the dreams of psychiatric patients, as our sample of the wider sample of dream studies, underscores a widespread neglect of methodological issues that serves to vitiate the findings of these and perhaps most dream studies. The suggestion that we have made little or no progress in answering the fundamental questions about dreams because of the sterility of our approach remains an open one, given the severe methodological limitations that have been reviewed. This is indeed unfortunate, as the more fundamental questions that we have about dream construction and dreaming's role in adaptation cannot be addressed by these studies. A more rigorous methodological approach and the systematic use of various study designs will be necessary before we dismiss dream research studies in answering our questions.

REFERENCES

1. Kramer M, Winget C, Roth T. Problems in the definition of the REM dream. In: Koella W, Levin P, editors. Sleep 1972. Basel (Switzerland): S. Karger; 1975. p. 149–56.
2. Chase M. The sleeping brain: perspectives in the brain sciences, vol. 1. Los Angeles (CA): Brain Information Services/Brain Research Institute; 1972. p. 247.
3. Pagel J, Blagrove M, Levin R, et al. Definitions of dream: a paradigm for comparing field descriptive specific studies of dream. Dreaming 2001;11:195–202.
4. Nagera H. Basic psychoanalytic concepts on the theory of dreams. New York: Basic Books; 1969. p.15.
5. Morris W. The American heritage dictionary of the English language. Boston: Houghton-Mifflin; 1969. p. 397.
6. Klinger E. Structure and functions of fantasy. New York: Wiley-Interscience; 1971. p. 51.
7. Malcolm N. Dreaming. New York: Humanities Press; 1959.
8. Erickson E. The dream specimen of psychoanalysis. J Amer Psychoanal 1954;2:5–56.
9. Taub J, Kramer M, Arand D, et al. Nightmare dreams and nightmare confabulations. Compr Psychiatry 1978;19:285–91.
10. Winget C, Kramer M. Dimensions of dreams. Gainscville (FL): University Presses of Florida; 1979. p. 6–21.
11. Kramer, M. The dream experience: a systematic exploration. New York: Routledge, Taylor and Francis Group; 2007.
12. Dennett D. Sweet dreams: philosophical essays on dreaming. Ithaca (NY): Cornell University Press; 2005. p. 227–50.
13. Ramsey G. Studies of dreaming. Psychol Bull 1953; 50:432–55.
14. Freud S. The interpretation of dreams. New York: Basic Books; 1955. p. 43.
15. Whitman R. Remembering and forgetting dreams in psychoanalysis. J Am Psychoanal Assoc 1983;11: 752–4.
16. Roth T, Kramer M, Trinder J. Volunteers versus nonvolunteers in dream research. Psychophysiology 1972;9:116.
17. Overton D. State-dependent retention of learned responses produced by drugs. Its relevance to sleep learning and recall. In: Koella W, Levine P, editors. Sleep 1972. Basel (Switzerland): S. Karger; 1973. p. 48–53.
18. Belicki K. Recalling dreams: an examination of daily variations and individual differences. In: Gackenbach J, editor. Sleep and dreams: a source book. New York: Garland; 1986. p. 187–206.
19. Kramer M, Winget C, Whitman R. A city dreams: a survey approach to normative dream content. Am J Psychiatry 1971;127:1350–6.
20. Webb W, Kersey J. Recall of dreams and the probability of stage 1-REM sleep. Percept Mot Skills 1967;24:627–30.
21. Snyder F. The physiology of dreaming. In: Kramer M, editor. Dream psychology and the new biology of dreaming. Springfield (IL): Charles C. Thomas; 1969. p. 7–31.
22. Kramer M, Whitman R, Baldridge B, et al. Patterns of dreaming: the interrelationship of the dreams of the night. J Nerv Ment Dis 1964;139:426–39.
23. Whitman R, Kramer M, Baldridge B. Which dream does the patient tell? Arch Gen Psychiatry 1963;8: 277–82.

24. Fox R, Kramer M, Baldridge BJ, et al. The experimenter variable in dream research. Dis Nerv Syst 1968;29:698–701.

25. Cartwright R, Kasniak A. The social psychology of dream reporting. In: Ellman S, Antrobus J, editors. The mind in sleep. 2nd edition. New York: Wiley; 1991. p. 251–64.

26. Piccione P, Thomas S, Roth T, et al. Incorporation of the laboratory situation in dreams. Sleep Res 1976; 5:20.

27. Schwartz J, Kramer M, Palmer T, et al. The relationship of personality factors to REM interruption diary recall of dreams. Sleep Res 1973;2:113.

28. Trinder, Kramer. Dream recall. Am J Psychiatry 1971; 128:296–301.

29. Kramer M, McQuarrie E, Bonnet M. Dream differences as a function of REM period. Sleep Res 1981;9:155.

30. Kramer M, Roth T, Czaya J. Dream development within a rem period. In: Koella W, Levin P, editors. Sleep 1974. Basel: S.Karger; 1975. p. 406–8.

31. Kramer M, Moshiri M, Scharf M. The organization of mental content in and between the waking and dreaming state. Sleep Res 1982;11:106.

32. Arand D, Kramer M, Czaya J, et al. Attitudes toward sleep and dreams in good versus poor sleepers. Sleep Res 1972;1:130.

33. Goodenough D, Lewis H, Shapiro A, et al. Dream reporting following abrupt and gradual awakenings from different types of sleep. J Pers Soc Psychol 1965;56:170–9.

34. Barber B. Factors underlying individual differences in rate of dream reporting. Psychophysiology 1969; 6:247–8.

35. Kramer M, Schoen L, Kinney L. Psychological and behavioral features of disturbed dreamers. Psychiatr J Univ Ott 1984;9:102–6.

36. Kramer M, Schoen L, Kinney L. The dream experience in dream disturbed Vietnam veterans. In: Van der Kolk B, editor. Post traumatic stress disorders: psychological and biologic sequellae. Washington, DC: American Psychiatric Press; 1984. p. 82–95.

37. Kramer M, Roth T. Dreams and dementia: a laboratory exploration of dream recall and dream content in chronic brain syndrome patients. Int J Aging Hum Dev 1975;6:179–82.

38. Herman J, Ellman S, Roffwarg H. The problem of N-REM recall re-examined. In: Arkin A, Antrobus J, Ellman S, editors. The mind in sleep: psychology and psychophysiology. Hillside (NJ): Erlbaum; 1978. p. 59–92.

39. Bonnet M, Alter J, Kramer M. Memory for events occurring during arousal from sleep. Sleep Res 1981;10:124.

40. Fiss H, Klein G, Bokert E. Waking fantasies following interruption of two types of sleep. Arch Gen Psychiatry 1966;14:543–51.

41. Goodenough D. Dream recall: history and current status of the field. In: Arkin A, Antrobus J, Ellman S, editors. The mind in sleep: psychology and psychophysiology. Hillside (NJ): Erlbaum; 1978. p. 113s–40s.

42. Goodenough D, Koulack D. Dream recall and dream recall failure: an arousal-retrieval model. Psychol Bull 1976;83:975–84.

43. Kramer M, Roth T. Dreams in psychopathologic patient groups: a critical review. In: Williams R, Karacan Ismet, editors. Sleep disorders, diagnosis and treatment. New York: John Wiley and Sons; 1978. p. 323–49.

44. Kramer M, Nuhic Z. A review of dreaming by psychiatric patients: an update. In: Pandi S, Ruoti R, Kramer M, editors. Sleep and psychosomatic medicine. New York: Taylor and Francis Group; 2007. p. 137–55.

Do Sleep Disorders Affect the Dreaming Process? Dream Recall and Dream Content in Patients with Sleep Disorders

Michael Schredl, PhD

KEYWORDS

- Sleep disorders • Dreaming
- Dream content • Dream recall

Dreaming, defined as mental activity that occurs during sleep,[1] is naturally closely related to sleep physiology.[2] So, the question arises as to whether or not the presence of a distinct sleep disorder alters dream recall or dream content.

This article reviews the studies investigating dreaming in patients with sleep disorders, such as insomnia, sleep apnea syndrome, narcolepsy, restless legs syndrome, and parasomnias. To understand the possible link between sleep disorders and dreaming, 3 theoretic frameworks are briefly introduced: the arousal-retrieval model of dream recall, the continuity hypothesis of dreaming, and the mind-body interaction during REM sleep.

DREAM RECALL: AROUSAL-RETRIEVAL MODEL

The arousal-retrieval model[3] hypothesizes that two steps are necessary for recalling a dream. For the first step, a certain amount of cortical arousal is necessary to transfer information (in this case, the dream content) from short-term into long-term memory. A period of wakefulness must follow the dream experience for the person to recall it because these storage processes do not occur during sleep. Once the dream is stored in long-term memory, the second step of the model, retrieval of the memory, takes place. Salience[4] and interference[5] can be integrated as factors that might affect retrieval of the information. A salient dream is more easily recalled and interference that occurs during retrieval impedes successful dream recall. Based on the repression hypothesis,[6] the model predicts that intense emotions might also reduce the chance of recalling the dream.

In persons without sleep disorders, frequency of nocturnal awakenings (see articles by Cory and colleagues[7] and Schredl and colleagues[8]) and low sleep quality (see articles by Lugaresi and colleagues[9] and Schredl and colleagues[10]) are associated with heightened dream recall frequency, supporting the importance of the first step of the arousal-retrieval model. Findings regarding the effect of cortical activation before awakening, as measured by an electroencephalogram (EEG), on the ability to remember the dream experience are conflicting (for overview, see article by Schredl[11]). Some studies found an increase in beta activity that was related to better dream recall[12,13] but others failed to find any correlation between EEG parameters of activation and dream recall.[11]

Findings regarding the effects of salience, interference, and repression—the second step of the arousal-retrieval model—are also conflicting (for overview, see article by Schredl[11]). For example,

Sleep laboratory, Central Institute of Mental Health, PO Box 12 21 20, Mannheim 68072, Germany
E-mail address: Michael.Schredl@zi-mannheim.de

Sleep Med Clin 5 (2010) 193–202
doi:10.1016/j.jsmc.2010.01.008

interference reduced dream recall under sleep laboratory conditions[5] but did not seem to be of importance in explaining the variance in home dream recall.[14] Similarly, dream salience was often not related to dream recall frequent.[15] Repression as a trait measure was not related to dream recall in most of the studies.[11] The empiric evidence only partially supports the arousal-retrieval model. In regard to sleep disorders, it could be predicted that sleep disorders accompanied by frequent nocturnal awakenings are associated with elevated dream recall frequency.

DREAM CONTENT: THE CONTINUITY HYPOTHESIS

Although Freud stressed the importance of day residues as constituents of dreams and linked many of his own dreams to his everyday experiences,[16] the term *continuity hypothesis* was formally introduced into dream research by Hall and Nordby.[17] The basic notion is that dreams reflect waking concerns and emotional preoccupations.[18] Schredl[19] proposed a more detailed model for the relationship between waking life experience and dream content that includes several factors that can modulate the probability of specific experiences, thoughts, and feelings from waking life being incorporated into subsequent dreams. The model includes the following factors: (1) exponential decrease of the incorporation rate of waking life experiences into dreams with elapsed time, (2) emotional involvement, (3) type of waking life experience, (4) personality traits, and (5) time of the night.

To test the continuity hypothesis, 2 different approaches are used: experimental manipulation and field studies. Although experimental studies (for example, that reported by De Koninck and Brunette[20]) have not found strong effects of presleep stimuli on dream content, field studies (for example, those reported by Schredl and Hofmann[21] and by Schredl and Piel[22]) demonstrate a relationship between waking experience and dream content. Emotional intensity of a waking life experience is directly related to the incorporation rate of this event into subsequent dreams, as confirmed by a diary study.[23] The empiric evidence reviewed by Schredl[19] indicates that the model is largely supported although systematic research is still lacking.

Regarding the dream content of patients with sleep disorders, it could be predicted that patients' waking life experiences (eg, stress levels and distress associated with the sleep disorder) would be reflected in their dreams (for example, the dreams include more negatively toned emotions).

DREAM CONTENT: THE MIND-BODY INTERACTION

Since the beginning of dream research in the sleep laboratory, researchers have studied whether or not the physiologic parameters, such as eye movements, heart rate, and EEG or electromyographic parameters, are related to the subjective experience of sleepers.[24] In 1892, Ladd[25] formulated the scanning hypothesis that states that the eye movements in REM sleep are directly related to gaze shift within the dream environment. Several studies[26,27] found empiric support by matching dream reports with the corresponding electrooculogram recordings. Herman and colleagues[28] pointed out the methodologic problems of this type of research, for example, the recall of every gaze shift within the dream or the standard eye movement measurement method, and concluded that there is a relationship between dream experience and eye movements of a sleeper but that the relationship is not close. For lucid dreaming, however, eye movements performed by a dreamer were clearly distinguishable from spontaneous eye movements.[2] Limb EEG recordings were matched to dreamed physical activity[29,30] and Hobson and colleagues[31] reported a relationship of short breathing pauses to dream content in healthy persons. For example, a dreamer reported—after being awakened from a REM period with a brief apnea—that he had been choked as part of a theater play. From a theoretic viewpoint, it is interesting to study patients with periodic limb movements or sleep apnea syndrome to test whether or not physiologic events, such as leg movements or breathing pauses, have an effect on dream content.

DREAMING AND SLEEP DISORDERS: OVERVIEW

Table 1 presents an overview of the studies investigating dreaming in patients with sleep disorders. Several topics have not been studied at all and, in some areas, only preliminary data (for primary hypersomnia and night terror/sleepwalking) or few studies (of insomnia, restless legs syndrome, sleep apnea, and narcolepsy) have been published. The REM sleep–associated parasomnias, nightmares and REM sleep behavior disorder (RBD), have been studied most extensively because dreams are at the core of the disorder. The research for each sleep disorder is reviewed.

Insomnia

Although a laboratory study including 26 patients with primary insomnia did not find differences in

Table 1
Dream recall, nightmare frequency/negative dream emotions, and dream content in patients with sleep disorders

Sleep Disorder	Dream Recall	Nightmares/ Negative Dream Emotions	Dream Content
Primary insomnia	↑[a]	↑	More problems
Restless legs syndrome	=[b]	=	—[c]
Sleep apnea syndrome	=	=	No breathing-related dreams
Narcolepsy	↑	↑	More bizarre and longer dreams
Primary hypersomnia	=	—	—
Night terrors/sleepwalking	=	↑	—
Nightmares	↑	↑	Being chased, falling, etc.
RBD	—	—	Aggressive dreams, gross body movements

[a] ↑, Heightened in patients compared with healthy controls.
[b] =, Comparable with healthy controls.
[c] —, Not studied.

the recall of visual dreams after experimental REM awakenings or non-REM (NREM) awakenings,[32,33] home dream recall was elevated in insomnia patients (N = 198) compared with healthy controls.[34] Because the group difference vanished when the frequency of nocturnal awakenings (questionnaire scale) was covaried in the statistical analysis, the idea that heightened dream recall frequency is due to the frequency of nocturnal awakenings is supported. This interpretation is supported by findings of positive correlations between frequency of nocturnal awakenings and dream recall frequency in healthy persons.[7,8,10] The heightened dream recall frequency seems plausible because the chance to recall a dream after awakening increases with the number of awakenings per night. In clinical practice, insomnia patients often report that they must have slept because they remembered dreams (ie, sleep state misperception [thinking that they are awake although the polysomnograhic record indicates a sleep stage] is smallest for REM sleep).[35]

Two studies[36,37] reported that persons with insomnia complaints report nightmares more often than patients without insomnia. Both samples, however, not only consisted of patients with primary insomnia but also included patients with other diagnoses (eg, depression). A recent study, including 295 polysomnographically diagnosed patients with primary insomnia, found more nightmares in this patient group compared with healthy controls.[38] Moreover, several studies[34,39–41] found

more negatively toned dreams in patients with insomnia. In addition, negative dream emotions correlated with the number of waking life problems.[34] Taking into account that stressors or major life events can trigger insomnia, these findings are in line with the continuity hypothesis of dreaming.

A small pilot study[42] that included 44 diary dreams of 6 insomnia patients did not find any differences in dream length, dream emotions, and problems occurring in the dreams when compared with the dreams of healthy controls. The dream series of one patient, however, reflected his waking life problems:

In the presence of my boss and several coworkers, I was unable to perform a repair job. After being verbally attacked by the boss, I told him that I would like to be placed in another department. Thinking about it, I regretted saying that because I felt that the job suits me and he is the one who is not qualified for the job because of his insufficient education.[42]

Ermann[43] studied the dream content of 26 insomnia patients obtained by REM awakenings in the sleep laboratory and after spontaneous awakenings during the night. The dreams of these patients more often contained negatives in self-description (eg, low self-esteem) and negatives in dream descriptions (eg, words, such as no or never, or references to something being missing). Schredl and colleagues[34] were able to confirm that negatives in self-description were more prominent in patients' dreams compared with the dreams of healthy controls. The other previously reported findings of negatives in dream descriptions and the reduced number of dream persons were not replicated, however. The patients reported longer dreams, fewer positive emotions, more problems within a dream, and more aggression and health-related themes than were present in the dreams of healthy controls (see **Table 1**). Moreover, the occurrence of waking life problems was significantly related to the occurrence of problems in their dreams ($r = 0.357$, $P<.005$, $N = 50$). Similarly, if the patients reported health problems, they dreamt about health-related issues more often ($r = 0.255$, $P<.05$, $N = 50$).

The content analytic findings support the continuity hypothesis to some extent because current stressors that might play a role in the cause of the insomnia are reflected in some of the patients' dreams (see previous dream example).

Restless Legs Syndrome

Schredl[44] studied dream recall frequency in a sample of 131 patients with restless legs syndrome. Dream recall frequency (questionnaire measure) was not elevated in comparison with healthy controls, a finding that would have been predicted by the arousal-retrieval model of dream recall because the frequency of self-reported nocturnal awakenings was markedly elevated in the patient group. The significant negative correlation between dream recall frequency and the index of periodic limb movements during sleep associated with arousals indicates that frequent arousals might interfere with dream recall or even with the dreaming process itself. Dream content analytic studies in patients with restless legs syndrome have not yet been published; but analyses of preliminary data obtained in the author's sleep laboratory did not show any content differences regarding dream leg movements compared with dream of healthy controls.

Sleep Apnea Syndrome

Questionnaire studies that applied a retrospective dream frequency scale with high retest reliability[45] have yielded mixed results. Whereas Schredl and colleagues[46] reported increased dream recall frequency in a sample of 44 sleep apnea patients, a second study[47] found lower dream recall frequency ($N = 309$) than in healthy controls. A third study[10] found no differences at all. This is in line with REM awakening studies[48–51] that report similar recall rates for patients and age-matched healthy controls

(64.2% versus 68.3%[48]; 51.5% versus 44.4%[49]). Furthermore, 3 studies[47,51,52] did not find any relationship between dream recall frequency and sleep apnea parameters, such as respiratory disturbance index (RDI) or oxygen saturation nadir. One explanation of this different finding regarding home dream recall might be provided by the study of Pagel and Shocknesse[53] showing that dream recall frequency in patients with sleep apnea was related to insomnia complaints.

In the nineteenth century, several researchers[54–57] hypothesized that nightmares are caused by a shortage of oxygen. de Groen and colleagues[58] reported a relationship between snoring, breathing pauses reported by the spouse, and nightmares in a sample of Dutch World War II veterans. In 2 student samples,[59,60] snoring was not related to nightmare frequency but the frequency of sleep reported breathing pauses. The first systematic study of nightmare frequency in sleep apnea patients ($N = 309$) found that, on average, nightmares occurred about once per month in the patient group, which was comparable with the mean of the healthy controls after correcting for age, gender, and overall dream recall frequency.[47] Moreover, nightmare frequency was not related to a RDI or the oxygen saturation nadir. Solely the presence of a psychiatric comorbidity, such as depression or anxiety disorder, was associated with heightened nightmare frequency in this patient group,[47] a finding that is in line with studies of psychiatric patients.[61] This was replicated in a second sample of sleep apnea patients ($N = 941$[52]). The findings indicate that sleep apnea patients do not suffer from nightmares caused by oxygen desaturation but by daytime stressors support the modern models of nightmare etiology.[62]

Regarding negative dream emotions, Gross and Lavie[50] reported that dreams were more negatively toned on nights with sleep apneas compared with nights with continuous positive airway pressure (CPAP) treatment. Carrasco and colleagues[49] reported a significantly increased number of violent and highly anxious dreams in 20 never-treated severe sleep apnea patients as compared with healthy controls and speculated as to whether or not a hyperactivation of the limbic system might explain this finding. More negatively toned dreams were also reported by 59 sleep apnea patients rating dreams recalled in the morning after a diagnostic night in the sleep laboratory.[51] Because intensity of negative emotions was not related to symptom severity (RDI or oxygen saturation nadir[46]), it might be speculated as to whether or not the more negatively toned dreams are explained by the continuity hypothesis (ie, they reflect patients' daytime problems engendered by daytime sleepiness).

In light of the findings regarding the mind-body interaction between dreaming and sleep physiology and the effects of internal and external stimuli on dream content, the question arises as to whether or not breathing-related dream content occurs in patients with sleep apnea. Despite some illustrative samples (discussed later), the results do not support this hypothesis. In 24 diary dreams of 5 sleep apnea patients,[42] in 44 REM and NREM awakenings dreams of 33 patients,[46] and in 34 REM awakening dreams of 20 patients,[49] no references to respiratory events were found. Gross and Lavie[50] and Schredl[51] found at least some evidence of breathing-related topics but the differences did not reach significance (eg, 2 out of 59 dreams in the report by Schredl[51]).

During the dream I felt tied up or chained. I saw thick ropes around my arms and was not able to move. I experienced the fear of suffocation without being able to cope with the situation. Powerlessness and also resignation came up. (Patient with sleep apnea, male, 39 years, RDI = 68.1 apneas per hour, maximal drop of blood oxygen saturation = 43%[51].)

I was diving without oxygen tanks and was gasping for breath. The way to the surface was far and I managed it just in time. After waking up I really gasped for breath. (Patient with REM sleep–associated sleep apneas, male, 39 years, RDI = 71.8, oxygen saturation nadir = 68%[47]).

Assuming that internal stimuli can affect dream content, it seems astonishing that apneas with such dramatic physiologic effects do not appear in dreams more frequently. One plausible explanation might be that the mind adapts to the slow progress of apnea severity over years. It would be necessary to conduct a study where participants wear a device (a full-face mask) that allows breathing to be blocked completely to investigate the effects of novel experienced respiratory pauses on dream content.

Schredl and colleagues[46] correlated RDIs with different dream characteristics and found a strong relationship with dream bizarreness ($r = -0.51$, $P<.005$, N = 33) (ie, high respiratory disturbance was associated with more realistic and less bizarre dreams). The finding of shorter than normal dream reports in sleep apnea patients[42,49] might point to a similar conclusion because research indicates that the duration of undisturbed REM sleep is related to dream report length.[26,63] The hypothesis that microarousals terminating breathing pauses might interfere with the dreaming process seems worthy of further study.

Effect of CPAP on dreaming

The treatment of sleep apnea syndrome with CPAP results in a dramatic change in sleep physiology (slow wave sleep rebound, REM rebound, and less fragmented sleep) in addition to reduction of the RDI.[49,64] A longitudinal study of the effects of CPAP on dreaming in a sample of 20 patients with severe sleep apnea (mean apnea-hypopnea index: 73.3) was performed by Carrasco and colleagues[49] They found a decrease in dream recall on the first CPAP night but an increase in dream length and positively toned dreams. These results can be interpreted as an effect of slow wave sleep rebound, which is associated with reduced dream recall and less fragmented sleep. The positively toned dreams, especially those found after 3 months and after 2 years of CPAP treatment, might be explained by the continuity hypothesis because CPAP treatment is often perceived as beneficial in patients with a severe sleep apnea syndrome. Thus, the possibility of increased limbic system activation during sleep in these patients as a cause of negatively toned dreams should be further examined.

Narcolepsy

A sample of 23 patients showed higher home dream recall frequency on a questionnaire measure.[65] Two REM awakening studies with 15 patients[66,67] and 17 patients[68] suffering from narcolepsy indicated that the percentage of recall after REM awakenings is high (about 90%) and comparable with the figures obtained from matched controls. The dreams of patients with narcolepsy have been described as vivid and often disturbing,[65,69–72] although Vogel[73,74] found equal proportions of negative and positive emotions in their sleep onset dreams. Alternatively, Mayer and colleagues,[75] analyzing the hospital records of 106 narcolepsy patients, found a prevalence rate of nightmares of 41.5% compared with about 5% in the general population. Vogel[73,74] and Fosse[66] reported that narcoleptic patients were more often aware of their state of consciousness during dreaming (ie, they knew that the dream experience was not real).

Dream content analysis of 14 dreams recorded by 8 patients during the laboratory diagnostic nights showed that the dreams were more bizarre than those of the control subjects.[65] A bizarre dream was reported by one female narcoleptic patient (age 20 years):

> I dreamt that I stepped out of the bright light of the lamp and slipped into another time period. I met my grandfather who I had never seen in my waking life and saw other persons from my hometown, much younger than today. With the help of friends I managed to travel back to the present time. I even brought some stuff from the past with me which my mother identified as her former belongings.[65]

To summarize, the deregulation of the REM sleep system underlying narcolepsy also manifests in cognitive changes, such as higher dream recall frequency and more negatively toned and bizarre dreams.

Primary Hypersomnia

Studying dream recall in patients with hypersomnia is of interest because several studies[76–78] have shown that longer sleep duration increases the probability to recall a dream. A sample of 99 patients diagnosed with primary hypersomnia, using 2 consecutive nights with polysomnography and a multiple sleep latency test during the day in-between, did not differ regarding dream recall frequency compared with healthy controls (manuscript in preparation). The author and colleagues speculated that the effect of longer sleep duration might be counteracted by sleep drunkenness that can be observed in some of these patients. How sleep inertia[79] (ie, cognitive deficits occurring in the brief time period after waking up) affects dream recall, however, has not yet been studied. In the author and colleagues' study, patients reported negatively toned dreams more often and their dreams were more often characterized by aggression and themes of illness. This can be seen as supporting the continuity hypothesis because patients with primary hypersomnia are often distressed by their daytime sleepiness.

Night Terrors/Sleepwalking

Night terrors and sleepwalking are NREM parasomnias and often occur together.[80] Broughton[81] coined the term disorders of arousal because the patients are partly awake (eyes open and seeing the surroundings) and partly asleep (no recollection and not able to carry out more sophisticated thinking or actions). Systematic study regarding dream recall and dream content outside the night terror or sleepwalking episodes has not been published. A small study of 28 patients diagnosed in the author's sleep laboratory showed that dream recall frequency was comparable with that of healthy controls. They reported more negatively toned dreams that correspond to the findings that NREM parasomnias co-occur with nightmares.[82] The negatively toned dreams might reflect stressors, which, alternatively, also increase the probability of nocturnal episodes in these patients.

Nightmares

Nightmares are defined as disturbing mental experiences that generally occur during REM sleep and that often result in awakening.[80] Nightmare frequency often correlates with dream recall frequency[83]; thus, nightmare sufferers show higher dream recall in general. By definition, these persons experience more negatively toned dreams than controls. The most common nightmare topics are being chased, falling, and death or injury of a close person.[84–86] Although there is a genetic disposition for nightmares,[87] the occurrence of waking life stressors is closely related to nightmare frequency.[83] This is in line with the continuity hypothesis of dreaming because nightmares at least partly reflect daytime stress.

REM Sleep Behavior Disorder

RBD is characterized by abnormal behaviors emerging during REM sleep usually manifesting as an attempted enactment of unpleasant, action-filled, and violent dreams.[80] By setting lesions in the brainstem areas responsible for muscle atonia in REM sleep, Jouvet[88] was able to observe acting-out behavior, such as prey catching or licking the fur. The loss of cells in the brainstem as a cause of RBD in humans is often a precursor to the development of a neurodegenerative disorder, such as Parkinson disease, Lewy body dementia, or multiple system atrophy. Systematic studies regarding dream recall have not yet been performed. Dream content—as discussed previously—in these patients is often described as violent and action packed (for example, see Fantini and colleagues[89]). Methodologic considerations, however, have to be taken into account when interpreting these findings. Fantini and colleagues'[89] study elicited most recent dreams, and it might be expected that patients report dreams that have been accompanied by body movements because they woke up due to injury or being awakened (ie, these patients report dreams that have been intense enough to break through the muscle atonia and thus these very intense dreams reflect the tip of the iceberg of their dream life in general). Diary studies and laboratory studies with REM awakenings have to be performed to determine whether or not normal dreaming is altered in these patients.

CLINICAL APPLICATIONS

The research findings discussed in this article can be useful for clinical practice in several ways. First, patients may report dreaming phenomena that they attribute to their sleep disorder or by which they are disturbed (eg, negatively toned dreams in patients with narcolepsy or heightened dream recall in insomnia patients). So it is useful for a sleep medicine specialist to know about altered dreaming in patients with sleep disorders to inform patients about these particular phenomena. Second, dream content may help to identify daytime stressors that are also of importance regarding the cause of the sleep disorder (eg, stress-related dreams in patients with insomnia or stress increasing nightmare frequency). Third, patients who are disturbed by their dreams might benefit from a brief intervention for coping with bad dreams and nightmares. Imagery rehearsal therapy,[90] which consists of 3 steps (record the dream, create a new ending for the dream, and rehearse a new dream over a 2-week period once a day) has been shown to be effective in several randomized controlled trials.[91] The therapeutic technique is so easy to understand that a brief handout outlining the basic principles might suffice to alleviate distress associated with dreaming. The use of lucid dreaming as a treatment of nightmares[92] might be especially well suited for patients with narcolepsy because studies reported frequent awareness that they are dreaming within the dream.

SUMMARY

Although the number of studies investigating dreaming in patients with sleep disorders is limited, overall the findings suggest that altered sleep physiology and other disorder-related variables have effects on dream recall and dream content in these patients.

The heightened dream recall frequency in insomnia patients supports the arousal-retrieval model of Koulack and Goodenough[3] (ie, that nocturnal awakenings play an important role in explaining differences in dream recall). Alternatively, studies in patients with sleep apnea and restless legs syndrome indicate that other factors, such as cognitive dysfunction or microarousals, play an important role. Thus, future studies should include cognitive measures and analyze the effects of microarousals[93] on dream recall. These findings will help to extend the present formulation of the arousal-retrieval model to account for the effects of sleep-related and cognitive variables.

Nightmares are not directly caused by a shortage of oxygen—because nightmare frequency is not elevated in sleep apnea patients—but the hypothesis put forward by Carrasco and colleagues[49] concerning hyperactivity of the limbic system during REM sleep in these patients is a topic for future research, especially if functional MRI studies can be achieved. Narcoleptic patients are suitable for such studies because they fall asleep quickly, often directly into a REM sleep episode.

Dream content studies indicate that physiologic processes, such as sleep apneas, are rarely reflected in dreams but support the continuity hypothesis[19] (eg, patients with more waking life problems dream more often about these problems). It would be useful to assess large samples of different sleep disorders patients to determine whether or not disorder-related symptoms, such as sleepiness, concentration problems, or lack of energy, are reflected in dream content. These findings could be combined with measures of distress to systematically test the model formulated by Schredl[19] (ie, to determine whether or not emotional involvement affects the probability of dreaming about a particular experience or symptom).

Because of the small number of studies in the field, additional research is needed to replicate and expand the findings reviewed in this overview. Such efforts would help to refine the arousal-retrieval, salience, and continuity hypotheses; deepen knowledge about the dreaming process; and provide further insight into the pathologies of sleep disorders patients that might benefit the patients.

REFERENCES

1. Schredl M, Wittmann L. Dreaming: a psychological view. Swiss Arch Neurol Psychiatr 2005;156:484–9.
2. Erlacher D, Schredl M. Do REM (lucid) dreamed and executed actions share the same neural substrate? Int J Dream Res 2008;1:7–14.
3. Koulack D, Goodenough DR. Dream recall and dream recall failure: an arousal-retrieval model. Psychol Bull 1976;83:975–84.
4. Cohen DB, MacNeilage PF. A test of the salience hypothesis of dream recall. J Consult Clin Psychol 1974;42:699–703.
5. Cohen DB, Wolfe G. Dream recall and repression: evidence for an alternative hypothesis. J Consult Clin Psychol 1973;41:349–55.

6. Freud S. Die Traumdeutung (1900). Frankfurt: Fischer Taschenbuch; 1987.

7. Cory TL, Orniston DW, Simmel E, et al. Predicting the frequency of dream recall. J Abnorm Psychol 1975; 84:261–6.

8. Schredl M, Wittmann L, Ciric P, et al. Factors of home dream recall: a structural equation model. J Sleep Res 2003;12:133–41.

9. Lugaresi E, Cirignotta F, Zucconi M, et al. Good and poor sleepers: an epidemiological survey of the San Marino population. In: Guilleminault C, Lugaresi E, editors. Sleep/wake disorders: natural history, epidemiology, and long-term evolution. New York: Raven Press; 1983. p. 1–12.

10. Schredl M, Bozzer A, Morlock M. Traumerinnerung und Schlafstörungen [Dream recall and sleep disorders]. Psychother Psychosom Med Psychol 1997; 47:108–16 [in German].

11. Schredl M. Dream recall: models and empirical data. In: Barrett D, McNamara P, editors. The new science of dreaming, vol. 2: content, recall, and personality correlates. Westport: Praeger; 2007. p. 79–114.

12. Rochlen A, Hoffmann R, Armitage R. EEG correlates of dream recall in depressed outpatients and healthy controls. Dreaming 1998;8:109–23.

13. Germain A, Nielsen TA, Khadaverdi M, et al. Fast frequency EEG correlates of dream recall from REM sleep. Sleep 1999;22(Suppl):131–2.

14. Schredl M, Montasser A. Dream recall: state or trait variable? Part I: model, theories, methodology and trait factors and part II: state factors, investigations, and final conclusions. Imagin Cogn Pers 1996–7;16: 181–210, 231–61.

15. Schredl M. The relationship between dream recall and dream content: negative evidence for the salience hypothesis. North Am J Psychol 2000;2:243–6.

16. Schredl M. Freud's interpretation of his own dreams in "The interpretation of dreams": a continuity hypothesis perspective. Int J Dream Res 2008;1: 44–7.

17. Hall CS, Nordby V. The individual and his dreams. New York: New American Library; 1972.

18. Domhoff B, Meyer-Gomes K, Schredl M. Dreams as the expression of conceptions and concerns: a comparison of German and American college students. Imagin Cogn Pers 2005–6;25:269–82.

19. Schredl M. Continuity between waking and dreaming: a proposal for a mathematical model. Sleep Hypnosis 2003;5:38–52.

20. De Koninck J, Brunette R. Presleep suggestion related to a phobic object: successful manipulation of reported dream affect. J Gen Psychol 1991;118: 185–200.

21. Schredl M, Hofmann F. Continuity between waking activities and dream activities. Conscious Cogn 2003;12:298–308.

22. Schredl M, Piel E. War-related dream themes in Germany from 1956 to 2000. Polit Psychol 2006; 27:299–307.

23. Schredl M. Factors affecting the continuity between waking and dreaming: emotional intensity and emotional tone of the waking-life event. Sleep Hypnosis 2006;8:1–5.

24. Schredl M. Body-mind interaction: dream content and REM sleep physiology. North Am J Psychol 2000;2:59–70.

25. Ladd GT. Contribution to the psychology of visual dreams. Mind 1892;1:299–304.

26. Dement WC, Wolpert EA. The relation of eye movements, body motility and external stimuli to dream content. J Exp Psychol 1958;44:543–53.

27. Roffwarg HP, Dement WC, Muzio JN, et al. Dream imagery: relation-ship to rapid eye movements of sleep. Arch Gen Psychiatry 1962;7:235–58.

28. Herman JH, Erman M, Boys R, et al. Evidence for a directional correspondence between eye movements and dream imagery in REM sleep. Sleep 1984;7:52–63.

29. Grossman WI, Gardner R, Roffwarg HP, et al. Relation of dreamed to actual movment. Psychophysiology 1972;9:118–9.

30. Gardner R, Grossman WI, Roffwarg HP, et al. The relationship of small limb movements during REM sleep to dreamed limb action. Psychosom Med 1975;37:147–59.

31. Hobson JA, Goldfrank F, Snyder F. Respiration and mental activity in sleep. J Psychiatr Res 1965;3: 79–90.

32. Ermann M, Peichl J, Pohl H, et al. Spontanerwachen und Träume bei Patienten mit psychovegetativen Schlafstörungen [Spontaneous awakenings and dreams in patients with psychophysiological sleep disorders]. Psychother Psychosom Med Psychol 1993;43:333–40 [in German].

33. Ermann M, Peichl J, Pohl H. Psychogene Schlafstörung als Traumstörung: Die Traumerinnerung bei Patienten mit psychovegetativen Schlafstörungen. In: Becker-Carus C, editor. Fortschritte der Schlafmedizin: Aktuelle Beiträge zur Insomnieforschung. Hamburg: LIT Verlag; 1994. p. 102–14.

34. Schredl M, Schäfer G, Weber B, et al. Dreaming and insomnia: dream recall and dream content of patients with insomnia. J Sleep Res 1998;7: 191–8.

35. Amrhein C, Schulz H. Selbstberichte nach dem Wecken aus dem Schlaf—ein Beitrag zur Wahrnehmung des Schlafes [Self reports after awakenings from sleep - a contribution to sleep perception]. Somnologie 2000;4:61–7 [in German].

36. Ohayon MM, Morselli PL, Guilleminault C. Prevalence of nightmares and their relationship to psychopathology and daytime functioning in insomnia subjects. Sleep 1997;20:340–8.

37. Hoffmann RM, Rasch T, Schnieder G. Fragebogen zur Erfassung allgemeiner Persönlichkeitsmerkmale Schlafgestörter (FEPS-I). Göttingen: Hogrefe; 1996.

38. Schredl M. Nightmare frequency in patients with primary insomnia. Int J Dream Res 2009;2:85–8.

39. Antrobus JS, Saul HN. Sleep onset: subjective behavioral and electroencephalographic comparisons. Waking Sleeping 1980;4:259–70.

40. Freedman RR, Sattler HL. Physiological and psychological factors in sleep-onset insomnia. J Abnorm Psychol 1982;91:380–9.

41. Strauch I, Maier B, Kaiser F. Developmental aspects of sleep onset insomnia in adolescents. In: Koella WP, Rüther E, Schulz H, editors. Sleep 1984. Stuttgart: Gustav Fischer Verlag; 1985. p. 386–8.

42. Schredl M. Traumerinnerungshäufigkeit und Trauminhalt bei Schlafgestörten, psychiatrischen Patienten und Gesunden [unpublished master thesis] University of Mannheim; 1991

43. Ermann M. Die Traumerinnerung bei Patienten mit psychogenen Schlafstörungen: Empirische Befunde und einige Folgerungen für das Verständnis des Träumens. In: Leuschner W, Hau S, editors. Traum und Gedächtnis: Neue Ergebnisse aus psychologischer, psychoanalytischer und neurophysiologischer Forschung. Münster: LIT Verlag; 1995. p. 165–86.

44. Schredl M. Dream recall frequency of patients with restless legs syndrome. Eur J Neurol 2001; 8:185–9.

45. Schredl M. Reliability and stability of a dream recall frequency scale. Percept Mot Skills 2004; 98:1422–6.

46. Schredl M, Kraft-Schneider B, Kröger H, et al. Dream content of patients with sleep apnea. Somnologie 1999;3:319–23.

47. Schredl M, Schmitt J, Hein G, et al. Nightmares and oxygen desaturations: is sleep apnea related to heightened nightmare frequency? Sleep Breath 2006;10:203–9.

48. Groß M. Dreams of patients with and without sleep apnea in the sleep laboratory. Israel Institute of Technology [Haifa: Research thesis] 1991.

49. Carrasco E, Santamaria J, Iranzo A, et al. Changes in dreaming induced by CPAP in severe obstructive sleep apnea syndrome patients. J Sleep Res 2006; 15:430–6.

50. Gross M, Lavie P. Dreams in sleep apnea patients. Dreaming 1994;4:195–204.

51. Schredl M. Träume und Schlafstörungen: Empirische Studie zur Traumerinnerungshäufigkeit und zum Trauminhalt von schlafgestörten PatientInnen. Marburg: Tectum; 1998.

52. Schredl M, Schmitt J. Dream recall frequency and nightmare frequency in patients with sleep disordered breathing. Somnologie 2009;13:12–7.

53. Pagel JF, Shocknesse S. Dreaming and insomnia: polysomnographic correlates of reported dream recall frequency. Dreaming 2007;17:140–51.

54. Waller J. Abhandlung über das Alpdrücken, den gestörten Schlaf, erschreckende Träume und nächtliche Erscheinungen. Frankfurt: Philipp Heinrich Guilhauman; 1824.

55. Strahl M. Der Alp, sein Wesen und seine Heilung. Berlin: Theod. Chr. Fr. Enslin; 1833.

56. Boerner J. Das Alpdrücken: Seine Begründung und Verhütung. Würzburg: Carl Joseph Becker; 1855.

57. Cubasch W. Der Alp. Berlin: Habel; 1877.

58. de Groen JHM, Op den Velde W, Hovens JE, et al. Snoring and anxiety dreams. Sleep 1993; 16:35–6.

59. Hicks RA, Bantista J. Snoring and nightmares. Percept Mot Skills 1993;77:433–4.

60. Schredl M. Snoring, breathing pauses, and nightmares. Percept Mot Skills 2008;106:690–2.

61. Schredl M, Engelhardt H. Dreaming and psychopathology: dream recall and dream content of psychiatric inpatients. Sleep Hypnosis 2001;3: 44–54.

62. Spoormaker VI, Schredl M, Van den Bout J. Nightmares: from anxiety symptom to sleep disorder. Sleep Med Rev 2006;10:19–31.

63. Dement WC, Kleitman N. The relation of eye movements during sleep to dream activity: an objective method for the study of dreaming. J Exp Psychol 1957;53:339–46.

64. Aldrich M, Eiser A, Lee M, et al. Effects of continuous positive airway pressure on phasic events of REM sleep in patients with obstructive sleep apnea. Sleep 1989;12:413–9.

65. Schredl M. Dream content in narcoleptic patients: preliminary findings. Dreaming 1998;8:103–7.

66. Fosse R. REM mentation in narcoleptics and normals: an empirical test of two neurocognitive theories. Conscious Cogn 2000;9:488–509.

67. Fosse R, Stickgold R, Hobson JA. Emotional experience during rapid-eye-movement sleep in narcolepsy. Sleep 2002;25:724–32.

68. Cipolli C, Bellucci C, Mattarozii K, et al. Story-like organization of REM-dreams in patients with narcolepsy-cataplexy. Brain Res Bull 2008;77:206–13.

69. Nixon OL, Pierce CM, Lester BK, et al. Narcolepsy: nocturnal dream frequency in adolescents. J Neuropsychiatr 1964;5:150–2.

70. Passouant P, Cadilhac J. Activite onirique et narcolepsie [Dream activity and narcolepsy]. J Psychol Norm Pathol 1967;64:171–87 [in French].

71. Roth B, Bruhova S. Dreams in narcolepsy, hypersomnia and dissociated sleep disorders. Exp Med Surg 1969;27:187–209.

72. Lee JH, Bliwise DL, Labret-Bories E, et al. Dream-disturbed sleep in insomnia and narcolepsy. J Nerv Ment Dis 1993;181:320–4.

73. Vogel GW. Studies in psychophysiology of dreams: III. The dream of narcolepsy. Arch Gen Psychiatry 1960;3:421–8.

74. Vogel GW. Mentation reported from naps of narcoleptics. Adv Sleep Res 1976;3:161–8.

75. Mayer G, Kesper K, Peter H, et al. Untersuchung zur Komorbidität bei Narkolepsiepatienten [Studying the comorbidity in patients with narcolepsy]. Dtsch Med Wochenschr 2002;127:1942–6 [in German].

76. Taub JM. Dream recall and content following extended sleep. Percept Mot Skills 1970;30: 987–90.

77. Schredl M, Fulda S. Dream recall and sleep duration: state or trait factor. Percept Mot Skills 2005; 101:613–6.

78. Schredl M, Reinhard I. Dream recall, dream length and sleep duration: state or trait factor. Percept Mot Skills 2008;106:633–6.

79. Tassi P, Muzet A. Sleep inertia. Sleep Med Rev 2000; 4:341–53.

80. American Academy of Sleep Medicine. The international classification of sleep disorders. (ICSD-2). Westchester: AASM; 2005.

81. Broughton RJ. Sleep disorders: disorders of arousal? Enuresis, somnambulism, and nightmares occur in confusional states of arousal, not in "dreaming sleep". Science 1968;159: 1070–8.

82. Schredl M, Blomeyer D, Görlinger M. Nightmares in children: influencing factors. Somnologie 2000;4: 145–9.

83. Schredl M. Effects of state and trait factors on nightmare frequency. Eur Arch Psychiatry Clin Neurosci 2003;253:241–7.

84. Garfield P. Your child's dreams. New York: Ballentine; 1984.

85. Schredl M, Pallmer R, Montasser A. Anxiety dreams in school-aged children. Dreaming 1996;6:265–70.

86. Zadra A, Duval M, Begin E, et al. Content analysis of nightmares. Sleep Suppl 2004;27:A64.

87. Hublin C, Kaprio J, Partinen M, et al. Nightmares: familial aggregation and association with psychiatric disorders in a nationwide twin cohort. Am J Med Genet 1999;88:329–36.

88. Jouvet M. What does a cat dream about? Trends Neurosci 1979;2:280–2.

89. Fantini ML, Corona A, Clerici S, et al. Aggressive dream content without daytime aggressiveness in REM sleep behavior disorder. Neurology 2005;65: 1010–5.

90. Krakow B, Zadra A. Clinical management of chronic nightmares: imagery rehearsal therapy. Behav Sleep Med 2006;4:45–70.

91. Wittmann L, Schredl M, Kramer M. The role of dreaming in posttraumatic stress disorder. Psychother Psychosom 2007;76:25–39.

92. Spoormaker VI, Van den Bout J. Lucid dreaming treatment for nightmares: a pilot study. Psychother Psychosom 2006;75:389–94.

93. Bonnet M, Carley D, Carskadon M, et al. EEG arousals: scoring rules and examples. Sleep 1992; 15:173–84.

Dream Content is Continuous with Waking Thought, Based on Preoccupations, Concerns, and Interests

G. William Domhoff, PhD

KEYWORDS

- Cognitive factors • Dream content • Gender differences
- Waking thought

According to age-old stereotypes that are constantly reinforced by stories in the mass media, the content of dreams is extremely bizarre, with little apparent rhyme or reason. The popular idea that dreams are mostly strange and otherworldly is reinforced by well-known freudian claims that they are full of disguised impulses and arcane symbolism. Bizarreness is also the dominant theme in one of the most publicly visible dream theories of recent decades, the activation-synthesis theory advocated by Hobson.[1] According to this theory, the unusual juxtapositions and themes in dreams are not caused by disguise or symbolism, but are the reaction of an ill-prepared forebrain to random activation that arises periodically from the brainstem because of the onset of rapid eye movement (REM) sleep. Hobson's theory allows for the fact that the forebrain can draw on thought patterns and memories developed in the waking state to impose a certain degree of coherence on these chaotic stimuli, which means that dreams can provide at least some psychologic information about the dreamer, but dreams are still said to be "cognitive trash."[2]

Is dream content really as strange and puzzling as the mass media and these rival dream theorists claim? In the past four decades dream researchers have applied the objective quantitative method called "content analysis" to large numbers of dream reports to answer this question. The methodology consists of four basic steps that extract systematic patterns from qualitative texts: (1) creating clearly defined categories that can be understood and applied in a reliable way by any investigator; (2) tabulating frequencies for the categories; (3) using percentages, ratios, or other statistics to transform raw frequencies into meaningful data; and (4) making comparisons with normative samples or control groups.

Based on this approach, content analysts have reached very different conclusions than either the freudians or activation-synthesis theorists. For example, the most comprehensive content analysis of adult dream content in the sleep laboratory, based on 635 dream reports collected from 58 young men and women over 250 nights in a series of investigations between 1960 and 1967, characterized a prototypical REM dream report as a "clear, coherent, and detailed account of a realistic situation involving the dreamer and other people caught up in very ordinary activities and preoccupations, and usually talking about them."[3] Overall, the investigators claimed that as many as "90% would have been considered

Department of Psychology, University of California, Santa Cruz, Santa Cruz, CA 95064, USA
E-mail address: domhoff@ucsc.edu

Sleep Med Clin 5 (2010) 203–215
doi:10.1016/j.jsmc.2010.01.010

credible descriptions of everyday experience."[4] Building on these laboratory findings, and large numbers of dreams written down in classrooms and in personal dream diaries, most content analysts have further concluded that a person's primary preoccupations, concerns, and interests are the main influence on dream content.[5]

This article summarizes the main findings that demonstrate these claims. It demonstrates that dream content is generally consistent over time once young adulthood is reached and that any changes parallel changes in waking concerns. It also shows that dream content in general is continuous with waking thought in a relatively straightforward manner that suggests dreams are enactments or dramatizations closely related to stories and plays in waking life. The article begins by comparing the dreams of men and women to show the ways in which waking gender differences in concerns and interests are expressed in dreams. It then presents findings on a potentially diagnostic difference between the dreams of mental patients and normal controls. Finally, it turns to discoveries with lengthy dream journals kept by a wide range of individuals; the general results with dream journals are illustrated using studies of a child molester and a normal middle-aged woman.

Although the focus of this article is on variability in dream content because that may be of greater potential use in clinical settings, it is important to note that this variability occurs within the context of considerable similarity in dream content in adults across the world. For example, a detailed study of characters and social interactions in 13 sets of dreams collected in small traditional societies by anthropologists in the first seven decades of the twentieth century reported many similarities.[6] Men dreamed more often about other men than they did of women, but women dreamed equally about men and women, as is the case for males and females from a very young age in the United States.[7,8] In addition, there were always more individual characters than group characters and more familiar than unfamiliar characters. The rate of aggressions per character was higher than the rate of friendly interactions per character with one exception, and physical aggressions were usually more frequent than nonphysical aggressions. Both men and women dreamers were more often victims than aggressors in aggressive interactions. Turning to large industrialized democracies, studies of dream reports from college students in Canada, the Netherlands, Switzerland, Germany, India, Japan, and the United States show more similarities than differences.[6,9]

Furthermore, at least 70% to 75% of dream reports collected outside the sleep laboratory involve everyday scenes and events, as shown in most detail in a study of the appearance of familiar people, commonplace leisure activities, and involvement in work, school, or politics in 95 dream reports from 37 German male college students and 246 dream reports from 98 German female college students.[10] The everyday nature of most dream content is seen in the fact that 75.2% of the women's dreams and 62.1% of the men's dreams had at least one instance of one of four categories of familiar characters; 42.3% of the women's dreams and 27.4% of the men's had at least one instance from one of five leisure-time categories; and 20.3% of the women's dreams and 29.5% of the men's dreams contained mentions of work, school, or politics. Overall, only 12.6% of the women's dreams and 20% of the men's had no instance of any of the previously mentioned categories. Similar findings have been reported for the dreams of young children and teenagers in the United States and Switzerland.[11–14]

METHODOLOGY: CONTENT ANALYSIS USING THE HALL–VAN DE CASTLE SYSTEM

Most of the findings reported in this article come from the Hall–Van de Castle coding system, the most comprehensive and widely used system of content analysis for dreams.[15] It was first outlined in the 1950s and then finalized in the 1960s for use in a large-scale comparison of dreams collected in the sleep laboratory and at home from 12 young men, which showed that laboratory dreams were as realistic as other laboratory studies had found and added that home dream reports are very similar to those collected in the laboratory.[16,17] The Hall–Van de Castle coding system consists of 10 general categories that make it possible to classify every element that appears in a dream report (eg, characters, social interactions, activities, misfortunes, emotions, settings, and objects). Most categories contain two or more subcategories. Characters, for example, consist of humans, animals, and mythical creatures; such factors as gender, relation to the dreamer, and age further subdivide the category for human characters.

The system rests on the nominal level of measurement because of problems of reliability and psychologic validity with rating scales.[18–20] Raw frequencies are analyzed using percentages and ratios called "content indicators" to correct for the varying length of dream reports from sample to sample and other problems that defeat many other systems for coding dream content. Because of the distortions and mistakes created by the use of parametric statistics with nominal data, skewed distributions, or nonrandom samples, especially when sample sizes are uneven, P values are determined using the formula for the significance of differences between two proportions, which has the added virtue of providing the same results as a 2×2 chi-square with data expressed in percentages.[21] Effect sizes are determined by the use of Cohen's h statistic,[22] which uses an arcsine transformation calculated for the two samples to correct for the fact that standard deviations cannot be computed for data expressed in percentages; h is roughly twice as large as a percentage difference, except at the tails of the distribution, where it is even larger. An h of 0 to 0.20 is small, an h of 0.21 to 0.40 is moderate, and an h over 0.40 is large in dream content studies.[6]

The Hall–Van de Castle coding system includes normative findings based on five dream reports from each of 100 American college men and 100 American college women, which provide the basis for cross-cultural comparisons and for finding individual differences in dream content. The animal percent (total animals divided by the total number of characters of any kind) provides a useful example of the findings produced by the system because it has great variation by age and culture. It is as high as 30% to 40% in young children, but only 6% for men and 4% for women in American society. It is as high as 30% in some hunting and gathering societies, and exceeds the American level in all of the dream samples collected by anthropologists in many different parts of the world.[6]

Studies using the Hall–Van de Castle system show that it usually takes 15 to 25 dream reports before patterns begin to appear and as many as 125 dreams before inferences about concerns and interests (based on blind analyses in which nothing is known beforehand about the dreamer) are regularly confirmed by the dreamer or people who know the dreamer well. Two factors account for the need for a relatively large number of dream reports for making accurate inferences: most dream elements appear in less than half of all dream reports and the differences between people's dreams are often small in magnitude, as demonstrated in a study that used randomization statistics to make tens of thousands of comparisons among random subsamples of varying sizes.[23]

This article also draws on findings using the search engine and output tables on DreamBank.net, a Web-based dream archive that contains 22,000 dream reports from individuals and groups, 16,000 in English and 6000 in German. The site includes a search engine that locates individual words, long strings of words, or phrases by means of Unix regular expressions, which are codes used for pattern matching in computer programming.[24] There is evidence that DreamBank.net searches produce results similar to those using the Hall–Van de Castle coding system.[25,26]

DIFFERENCES BETWEEN MEN AND WOMEN

The dreams of men and women in the United States are similar in several ways, such as the same percentage of dreams with at least one aggression, or one friendly interaction, or one misfortune, and they have the same percentage of high negative emotions (80% of all the emotions in men and women's dreams are anger, apprehension, sadness, or confusion). They also show several gender differences that seem to parallel gender differences in waking life, however, which is evidence for an emphasis on concerns and interests in understanding dream content. For instance, there is a higher percentage of physical aggressions in men's dreams and a higher percentage of rejections and exclusions in women's dreams, which parallels the waking finding that boys engage in more physical aggression than girls and that girls are more likely to engage in "social aggression" (eg, exclusion, rejection, and criticism).[27] Differences in the activities and objects categories seem to parallel differences in the general waking concerns of men and women. For example, men's dreams have more physical activities and women are more likely to be engaged in conversations. There are more appearances of tools and cars in men's dreams, and more appearances of clothing and household items in women's dreams.[15] The pattern of similarities is presented in **Fig. 1**, which is based on differences on the effect size statistic h.

Similar gender differences emerged from the study of commonplace events in the dreams of German college students. The women's dreams more frequently involved familiar characters and everyday leisure-time activities than those of the men, but the men's dreams were more likely to have mentions of work, school, or politics, or to contain no commonplace activities.[10]

DIFFERENCES BETWEEN MENTAL PATIENTS AND NORMATIVE FINDINGS

There have been many studies of dream content in various psychiatric populations over the past 100

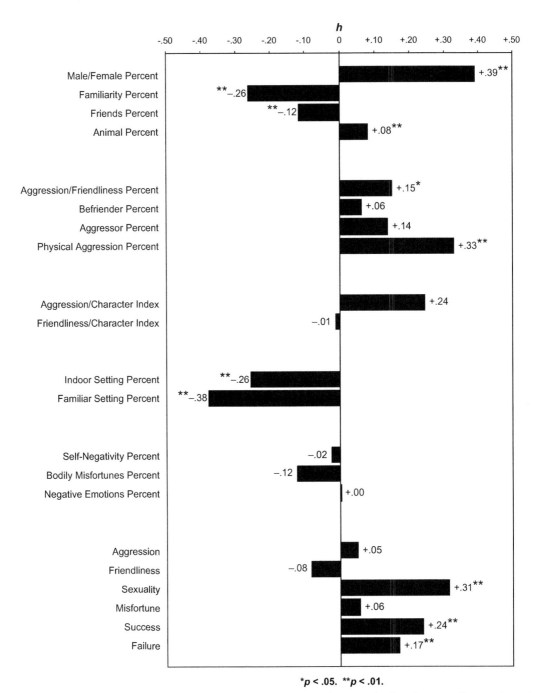

*p < .05. **p < .01.

Fig. 1. The *h*-profile for the Hall–Van de Castle male normative sample, using the female normative sample as the baseline.

years, but most of them are anecdotal in nature, use untested coding systems, or include only small numbers of patients, so there are few consistent findings. It is likely that variations from hospital to hospital in how patients are diagnosed and classified, the collection of dream reports from patients in different phases of their illness, and the possible effects of medication and hospitalization on both dream content and the ability to provide full and accurate dream reports also contribute to this inconsistency in findings.[28,29] Moreover, the most systematic study of differences between mental patients and the Hall–Van de Castle norms suggested very few differences, except on the important issue of friendly interactions. The study was based on 211 dream reports collected from 50 male patients, who were grouped into four diagnostic categories: 5 patients who were both schizophrenic and alcoholic, 20 patients who were schizophrenic, 15 patients who were alcoholics, and 10 patients with a variety of other diagnoses. The dream reports of the four groups were compared with each other and with the Hall–Van de Castle male norms for characters, social interactions, success and failure, misfortune and good fortune, and eating and drinking. Most of the differences among the patient groups were few and unrevealing (eg, dream reports from schizophrenics were shorter, and there were more instances of drinking alcohol and fewer sexual interactions in the alcoholics' dream narratives).

There was one potentially useful difference between the dreams of the 50 patients as a whole and the Hall–Van de Castle norms: a very low rate of friendly interactions, especially with women.[30] The finding is of interest because a similar low rate of friendliness also was the most striking outcome in a study of 27 hospitalized female patients, 15 of whom suffered from schizophrenia and 12 from other types of psychoses.[31] The same result is reported in a study of female outpatients who suffered from high anxiety states, and findings in a comparison of dream reports from depressed and schizophrenic patients studied in the laboratory revealed a lack of friends in patient dreams and a low rate of friendly interactions.[32,33] There have been no systematic studies of mental patients' dreams in recent decades, but a lack of friendly interactions in dreams may be the most promising diagnostic sign to examine in future studies.

STUDIES OF INDIVIDUAL DREAM JOURNALS

Dream journals, kept by a small number of people from all walks of life for varying reasons, have standing as a form of personal document long recognized in psychology as possessing the potential to provide new insights.[34,35] They are valued as "nonreactive" measures that have not been influenced by the purposes of the investigators who later analyze them. That is, they do not suffer from the "demand characteristics" that can be a confounding factor in many types of experiments in the psychologic sciences and medicine, including dream research. The findings with nonreactive archival data, such as dream journals, are considered most persuasive when they lead to the same conclusion even though the various journals have different types of potential biases because

of the differing motivations and purposes of the journal keepers.[36]

Quantitative analyses of numerous individual dream series over a period of five decades reveal that dream content is generally consistent for most individuals over months, years, and decades.[6] Even more important for this article, inferences from such studies based on blind analyses of the results reveal that most dream content is continuous with waking concerns and interests, as seen especially in the frequency with which the main people in the dreamer's life appear and in the way in which they are portrayed in social interactions (eg, aggressive, friendly, unresponsive). There are also clear indications of the dreamer's primary waking interests (eg, music, sports, traveling). Two detailed case studies, one based on the dreams of a child molester, one based on the dreams of middle-age normal adult, are used to demonstrate these points in detail, but there are other cases that can be drawn on, including a comparison of the dreams of Freud and Jung.[6,37–39]

It is necessary, however, to temper these generalities about continuity in three ways. First, the continuity is not with day-to-day events, but with general concerns. Three studies that tried to match detailed waking reports of daily concerns with dream reports, two based on REM awakenings and one based on morning recall at home, found that blind judges could not reliably match records of daily concerns or events with dream content. The content of the dreams often revolved around daily life, such as family, friends, and school, but if the actual events of the day were incorporated in any specific way, it was not understandable to independent raters.[40–42]

Secondly, the continuity usually is with both thought and behavior, but sometimes it is only with thought. For example, an analysis of a dream series with over 1000 dream reports from an engineer in his early 30s showed that sexuality in dream reports is not always accompanied by waking behavior related to the same activities as occurred in the dreams. Over the course of a 3-year period, the dreamer had sexual relations in his dreams with 38 different female characters, most of them women he knew and to whom he felt attracted in waking life. In waking life, however, he had not had intercourse with any of these women. Instead, the continuity was with his waking sexual fantasies, which were accompanied by masturbation once or twice each day.[6,39] Third, not all dream elements are continuous with waking concerns and interests, as shown in one of the dream series discussed in this section.

THE DREAMS OF A CHILD MOLESTER

An unusual opportunity to examine the degree to which dream content relates to waking preoccupations developed when a child molester in his mid-30s, imprisoned in a mental institution for sex offenders, revealed to one of the clinical psychologists who worked with him that he had written down 1368 dream reports over a period of years for his own personal interest, many of them on paper bags and laundry lists.[6,43] A complete Hall–Van de Castle coding of the dream reports revealed that he differed from the norms in only a few ways, but most of those differences turned out to be continuous with his waking thoughts or behavior. In particular, there were many unusual features in the character patterns in his dream reports, with his mother appearing 4 times more often than would be expected from the norms, and his sister appearing 10 times more often. There was no mention, however, of his father.

Beyond female family members, he dreamt primarily of unknown males and unknown females. The percentage of characters that were friends of the dreamer was only 9%, far below the normative figure of 31% for males, and there was an especially low incidence of female friends and acquaintances. As for the males who were known to him, they were usually his fellow inmates, not friends of long standing. The child molester was not unusually low on friendly interactions, however, because of his generally positive interactions with his mother and sister in his dreams, but also because he often befriended or helped children and teenagers.

The child molester had a typical number of dreams with at least one sexual thought or interaction, but his sexual dreams differed from those of other men in terms of the variety of characters with whom he was erotically involved and the types of interactions that occurred. Whereas heterosexual men have erotic encounters almost exclusively with peer females, he was involved in or witnessed sexuality in his dreams with men and women, and children and adults. He was also unusual in the range of sexual acts in which he engaged. In addition, his dream reports contained more sexual fantasies and less sexual intercourse than the male norms.

These dream findings fit with the reality of his waking life, where he was very dependent on his highly controlling mother and his supportive sister, whom he reported were the two most positive influences in his life. His father, often absent in his early years, was pushed out of the house by the patient's mother when the inmate-patient was 12 and died a few years later. He had no friends and preferred to be around children. As in his dreams, he had had sex with other males and at least once with an animal. His main sexual outlet, however, was the same compulsive voyeurism present in his dream reports. He wrote that he had always had "a morbid yet fascinating curiosity about the female genitals."[6] In his teenage years and early adulthood, his child molesting did consist primarily of looking at children's genitals, but later it included fondling on several occasions and exposure of himself at least once, which is why he was sentenced to the prison hospital for sex offenders.

There were also some informative differences between the dream content and his waking behavior. Although he masturbated frequently in his dreams, leading to the inference that he was a compulsive masturbator in waking life, he reported that he was able to refrain from masturbation for weeks at a time because he thought it was wrong and often felt depressed afterward. He used meditation and an interest in spirituality to help him control this urge, suggesting that an analysis of dream content may not always reveal how people actually deal with their desires in waking life.

THE DREAMS OF A MIDDLE-AGE WOMAN

The most comprehensive study of a dream series undertaken to date is based on 3116 dreams over a 20-year period from a normal woman who began writing them down for her own interest when she was in her early 30s; the original study was later supplemented with several word-string analyses of another 1138 dreams over a 5-year.[21] The dreams were coded using the Hall–Van de Castle system by researchers who knew nothing about her. The dreamer was interviewed for a 2-day period by this author to pose questions based on the blind analyses of the dream reports. He also interviewed four of her close women friends to have independent information on key issues in the event of any disagreements between inferences drawn from the dream codings and what the dreamer reported in reaction to the inferences (in this case there turned out to be no disagreements).

Born in the 1940s and raised in a small town, the dreamer was the oldest of four children, with a brother 2.7 years younger, a second brother 4.7 years younger, and a sister 6 years younger. Both of her parents earned college degrees at a small denominational college and worked all their lives in education and social work. The dreamer was an average high school student who married after 1 year of college and had three daughters in the space of 4.5 years. She earned a bachelor of arts degree in her mid-20s from a state college and divorced her husband at age 30, when her daughters were 7, 4.5, and 2.5 years of age. She left her daughters with her ex-husband and returned to her home state, where she earned a master of arts degree in a helping profession and worked in a community college setting for several years. She had several boyfriends after her divorce and never remarried. She became involved in local theater productions as an actress and director. She developed a strong interest in dreams and participated in dream groups.

As in previous studies, most of her dream content was consistent over the 25-year period. For example, at least 1 of the 13 main people in her life (parents, exhusband, three siblings, three children, granddaughter, and three best friends) appear in 33.6% of the dreams in the first set of dreams and 35.1% of the second set. Her continuing interest in theatrical productions (as a writer, actor, and producer) is reflected in the fact that 4.9% of the dreams in the first set contained one of several terms related to this activity, as compared with 5.2% for the second set. She was also consistent in the emotions expressed in her dreams, as shown in an analysis using lengthy word strings that relate to each of the five emotions that are coded in the Hall–Van de Castle coding system: (1) anger, (2) apprehension, (3) sadness, (4) confusion, and (5) happiness.[26] As displayed in **Table 1**, the percentages for each category of emotions are very similar for the two sets and also for the percentage of dreams with at least one emotion of any type.

The strikingly different patterns of social interactions with individual family members and close friends in the dreams correspond with her conceptions of these people and her relations with them in waking life. For example, the most frequently appearing character in her dreams is her mother, who is also her most important preoccupation in waking life. She appears in 239 of the first 3116 dream reports, or 7.7% of the total, which supports the repeated finding that the frequency of the appearance of a person or activity in a dream series reveals the intensity of waking concern with that person or activity. In addition, the dreams portray a highly conflicted relationship. This is shown by the fact that the aggressions per character ratio with her is 0.70, well above the dreamer's average of 0.32 for all characters in a random sample of 250 of her first 3116 dream reports (**Table 2**, where the random sample is labeled the "baseline 250). The aggression-friendliness percent in their social interactions (the total number of aggressions divided by the total number of aggressions plus the total number of friendly interactions) is 72%, which is well above the dreamer's normative figure of 49%. This aggression-friendliness percent is consistent over the entire series, as shown when the dreams are divided into thirds.

These findings reflect the way in which she describes her mother and her relationship with her in waking life:

My mother is an angry, isolating person, and she also has good things too, don't get me wrong. But she and I have had a personality clash as long as I can remember. I feel that she keeps herself so distant that I didn't feel I was getting nurturing mother love. I told one of my women friends that the love of my mother is like carrying a barbed blue baby blanket, you know, with barbs in it. It's supposed to be soft and cuddly and loving, but in fact, she was sharp and critical and negative and physically distant.

The dreamer said she had a more positive attitude toward her father, however, a claim that was corroborated by her friends. He appeared in 213 dream reports, second only to her mother. As shown in **Table 2**, the aggressions per ratio with him was 0.36, not far above her normative figure with all characters, and the friendliness per character ratio was 0.37, once again slightly above her normative figure. The aggression-friendliness percent with him was 50%. Although there is nothing striking about her relationship with him, it is dramatically different from her relationship with her mother.

The dreamer's middle daughter was almost as problematic for her as her mother. This daughter was 4.5 years old at the time of the divorce, and

Table 1
The consistency of emotion in two halves of the dream series using key word searches

	Anger %	Apprehension %	Sadness %	Confusion %	Happiness %	Any Emotion %
Set 1 (N = 3116)	18.3	30.8	10.3	11.3	13.5	56.1
Set 2 (N = 1138)	15	31.8	9.8	14.5	15.5	57.8

Table 2
The dreamer's social interactions with significant people in her life, compared with the baseline 250 sample

	N	Aggression-Characters Index	Friendliness-Characters Index	Aggression-Friendliness %	Aggressor %	Befriender %
Baseline 250	884	0.33	0.32	49	50	53
Mother	239	0.70	0.27	72	46	48
Father	213	0.36	0.37	50	47	42
Oldest daughter	81	0.51	0.65	44	73	77
Middle daughter	165	0.92	0.52	64	79	70
Youngest daughter	83	0.36	0.81	31	63	61
Favorite brother	97	0.23	0.69	25	59	60
Friend Ginny	96	0.26	0.89	23	52	53
Friend Lucy	59	0.39	0.63	38	78	78

was the most upset by it of the three children. At age 14 she ran away from her father's home and came to live with her mother. She did poorly in school, could not hold on to a job, and suffers from severe psychologic problems. She had a daughter of her own when she was a teenager and soon left her to the dreamer to raise. She still returns to live with the dreamer from time to time. The dreamer worries about her constantly, and between them there is great tension.

This daughter appears in 165 dream reports. The aggressions per ratio is 0.92, even higher than with the mother, and the friendliness per character ratio is also very high at 0.52, well beyond the dreamer's average for all characters. Taken together, these two ratios show that between them there is a high rate of interaction. The aggression-friendliness percent is 64%, with the dreamer initiating 79% of the aggressive interactions and 70% of the friendly interactions, far above her averages for all characters. These indicators provide an accurate summary of how she conceives of their relationship.

By contrast, she dreams only half as often of her oldest and youngest daughters, who adjusted to the divorce better, went to school in their father's home state, saw their mother primarily during summer vacations, and live normal adult lives. The aggression-friendliness percents, 44% with the older daughter and 31% with the younger daughter, show that she has more friendly than aggressive interactions with both of them, which reflects her more positive relationship with them. As with the middle daughter, the dreamer is more likely to be the initiator of both aggressive and friendly interactions.

The dream reports also capture her positive relationships with the favorite people in her life. For example, she has great affection for the brother closest to her in age, who appears in 97 dream reports in the first set, which is one more than the total for her other two siblings combined. The aggression-friendliness percent with him is 25%, almost the mirror opposite of her interaction pattern with her mother. Positive patterns are also apparent with two women friends, but there are differences on some indicators, which reflect her different pattern of interaction with each of them. The dreamer met her closest friend of long standing, Ginny, when she returned to college for her masters degree. Ginny appears in 96 dream reports and has an aggression-friendliness percent of 23%, the most positive balance with any dream character. The comradely nature of their relationship is seen in the fact that they are equally likely to initiate friendly or aggressive interactions.

She met another close friend, Lucy, when Lucy was a student at the community college where the dreamer worked. The dreamer is the big sister in this relationship, giving Lucy instructions, helping her, and becoming annoyed when Lucy is late or resisting direction. This pattern is reflected in the fact that the dreamer initiates 78% of the many friendly interactions between them and 78% of the relatively few aggressive interactions.

As revealing as these findings are, they only scratch the surface of what it is possible to learn about people's conceptions and concerns from studying long dream journals. This claim is now demonstrated on the basis of in-depth studies of two subseries within this dream series. The first concerns her exhusband, whom she still bitterly disliked and could not think about without becoming upset for nearly 20 years. This subseries reads like a replay of her worst fears and grievances. The second subseries is about a man with whom she developed an infatuation for many years after her divorce and after she had not been dating anyone for several years. Because she had no romantic relation with this man, who did know about her feelings, all of the events in this subseries are completely from her imagination.

The Exhusband Dreams

The dreamer first met Howard, her future husband, when they were in high school, but they both had other love interests at the time. They became involved when he returned for the summer after his first year of college and they married after a year-and-a-half courtship. She remembers Howard from their years of marriage as a person who was insensitive to her need for tenderness and expression of feeling, as a person who just wanted sex. She believed that their sexual interactions sometimes felt more like rape than seduction.

Howard appears in 196 dreams, surpassed only by her mother, father, and middle daughter in the frequency of his appearances. These dreams have a fairly regular structure. They usually start with the dreamer noticing that Howard is back, causing her considerable apprehension or annoyance. At the outset he is often seeking reconciliation, although on occasion she is the one who is thinking about the possibility of getting back together. As the dream unfolds, Howard usually tries to initiate a sexual interaction through a touch or a kiss, but the dreamer is either hesitant or repulsed. Sometimes she is tempted, but then changes her mind.

Toward the end of the series, the Howard dreams seem to become somewhat more benign. In one or two dreams, she even entertains the idea of reconciliation, an idea for which there was no basis in her or his waking reality and which she did not think about in waking life. This impression of a change in the tone of the Howard dream reports is borne out by the large decline in the aggression-friendliness percent when the dreams about him are divided into four chronologic segments; there are proportionately more friendly interactions in the later years. This result is shown in **Table 3**. The dreamer' reflections on her feelings about Howard in my interview with her in March, 2000, parallel the main themes in the dreams.

Overall, the dreams about Howard are a classic example of the tendency to repeat long-standing themes, especially negative ones, in a dream series.[44] It is as if these themes are embedded in the vigilance and fear system centered in the amygdala and surrounding areas, and are subject to reactivation under circumstances that cannot be determined with the information that is available for this study. Moreover, these repetitive patterns seem to persist even though the dreamer believes she has gained greater perspective on her failed marriage in waking life. This belief is supported in the interviews with her friends, who noted that she talked about him less and expressed less anger than in the past. Perhaps dreams express past preoccupations and concerns even when there is a decline in those preoccupations in waking thought; perhaps waking thought may change more, or more quickly, than dreams change.

Dreams of a Failed Infatuation

Several years after she had dated anyone regularly, the dreamer met a man, Derek, whom she found very attractive. They had a common circle of friends and a mutual interest in the theater and dreams. Later they happened to be in the same playwriting and dream-sharing groups. Derek is 12 years younger than the dreamer and did not seem interested in more than a casual friendship in group settings, which she basically understood. Nonetheless, she became very infatuated with him and entertained the hope of a romantic relationship.

Derek appears in 43 dream reports during the time period covered by the systematic analysis. Overall, the dreams have a very high rate of

Table 3 Dreams about Howard: changes in the aggression-friendliness percent over time					
	Baseline Aggression-Friendliness %	1st Segment %	2nd Segment %	3rd Segment %	4th Segment %
Aggression-friendliness %	49	57	59	61	34

friendly and sexual interactions, and a low rate of aggressions, especially physical aggressions, as shown in the *h*-profile in **Fig. 2**. This *h*-profile compares dreams concerning Derek with dreams with Howard in them, using the results with the random sample of 250 of her dreams as the baseline. The contrast is dramatic and reflects her completely opposite feelings for the two men.

Thirteen of the first 16 dream reports concerning Derek contain sexual or intimate physical interactions with him. These early sensual dreams are in general very positive and full of anticipation, but they also express her fear that he does not care about her, and in one dream he even chases her after he has an orgasm. As the dreamer comes to accept that the relationship is not going to

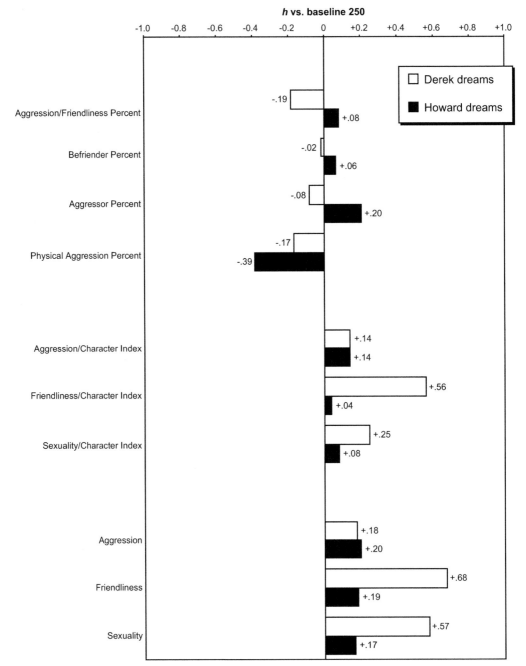

Fig. 2. An *h*-profile of dreams of Derek and Howard, compared with the baseline 250 sample.

become a romantic one, her sexual interactions with him in the dreams become less frequent. She also has dreams in which she is angry with him or jealous that he is having sex with someone else. About a month after she broke off their friendship because of her feelings of frustration, she had a dream in which she was upset because he was with another woman. Later she had a dream that implied they are still friends, even though she has not seen him in months. He then gradually disappeared from her dream life.

This subseries is striking for the fact of sexual intercourse and other sexual intimacies that have no correspondence to her waking reality. They are clearly wishful dreams. They are continuous with her waking hopes, but not with her waking life. They also dramatize the fact that he had no interest in a romantic relationship with her. Unlike the Howard subseries, however, they do decline greatly in frequency once she thinks about him less often in waking life.

Theater Dreams

It appeared from reading through the first several dozen dreams in this series that the dreamer has a strong interest in theatrical performances, whether as an actor, singer, or director. When a word string containing all relevant theater-related terms was entered into DreamBank.net, it retrieved 77 dream reports in which she is auditioning for, taking part in, or directing a theatrical production. This large number of theater dreams is continuous with her waking interests. She acts and sings in productions, some of which she writes herself. She also very much enjoys directing theatrical performances.

In half of the theater dreams where she is involved as a performer or director, she portrays herself as giving an excellent performance. It is clear from these positive theater dreams that the dreamer has, or once had, very high hopes and ambitions. She would very much like to be in the public limelight as an esteemed artistic figure. This inference of great ambition was supported in an interview with one of her friends with whom she often performs. An equal number of the theater dreams, however, contain rejections and misfortunes. She does not win the part, or people leave as she is about to perform. She misses a rehearsal, cannot find the theater, nearly falls off the stage, or forgets her lines or is afraid she will forget them. These negative events are consistent with two of her waking concerns in regard to her public performances. First, she is indeed afraid she will forget her lines, as attested to by both her and her friends. Second, she does believe she is

often ignored or unappreciated, a point that is stated most frankly by two of her friends.

Just as her dreams featuring significant people in her life enact the nature of her relationships with them, the theater dreams seem to be variations on a few of her major concerns about artistic performances. These concerns are the "themes" that are acted out to varying degrees in each dream relating to the theater and performances. That is, each individual dream can be seen as a specific instance from which generic information about her interests and concerns can be extracted.

Dream Elements that are not Continuous

Although this dream series demonstrates the large degree of continuity between dream content and waking concerns, there are some elements in it that are not continuous with her waking life. For example, she has several dreams about cats and kittens, but especially kittens that are neglected, deformed, or starving. The appearance of cats fits with her interest in cats in waking life, but contrary to the expectation of continuity, she does not worry about the health of cats, of which she has several, in waking life; nor does she fear that they might starve or be neglected.

Unlike kittens, horses are portrayed in a very positive light in the dream reports. She has 24 dreams in the overall series where she is riding a horse. In all of these dreams, she portrays herself as an excellent rider. Taken together, these dreams give the impression that she learned to ride as a child and likes horses, but this is not the case. Moreover, she was afraid of horses and had never ridden one alone; nor does she express any waking interest in riding a horse.

There is also a lack of continuity in relation to her use of guns and rifles in her dreams. There are 33 dream reports in the overall series in which she is holding or shooting a gun, always with confidence. She fixes and reloads guns, kills dangerous animals, and fights off human attackers. These positive dream actions led to the inference that she might have learned to shoot guns as a child and still enjoys doing so. That inference, however, proved to be incorrect; nor does she entertain any waking fantasies concerning guns or shooting.

Dreams that provide an exception to the basic finding of continuity with waking thoughts and concerns are valuable because they might help in developing a better understanding of dream meaning. Perhaps some dreams have metaphoric meaning, as freudian theory claims, or are fanciful adventure stories, such as her horse-riding and gun-shooting dreams. Perhaps they may reveal the limits of the conceptual systems available for dreaming during sleep, as activation-synthesis theory argues.

SUMMARY

This article highlights findings on the factors that seem to have the largest impact on dream content. Once people are young adults, their dreams are most strongly influenced by gender and individual differences, as seen in the normative comparisons of men and women and in the two illustrative case studies. Mental health status also may be a factor, but little progress has been made in understanding the dream content of psychiatric patients beyond the lack of friendly interactions because of the difficulties of doing systematic research with this population.

Building on the gender and individual-difference findings, this article shows that there is a more general and psychologically interesting factor that shapes dream content: the life experiences that generate each person's mix of preoccupations, concerns, and interests. It is these cognitive factors that make dreams a highly unique expression of how a person understands his or her own world. The intensity of interests is revealed by the frequency with which people and activities appear, and the way in which those people and activities are regarded is revealed by the varying ways in which they are portrayed. Dreams are a perceptual embodiment and dramatization of a person's thoughts, an fMRI of the mind at night. They are the quintessential cognitive simulation because they are experienced as real while they are happening.

REFERENCES

1. Hobson JA. The dreaming brain. New York: Basic Books; 1988.
2. Hobson JA. Dreaming: an introduction to the science of sleep. New York: Oxford University Press; 2002.
3. Snyder F. The phenomenology of dreaming. In: Madow L, Snow L, editors. The psychodynamic implications of the physiological studies on dreams. Springfield (IL): Thomas; 1970. p. 124–51.
4. Snyder F, Karacan I, Tharp V, et al. Phenomenology of REM dreaming. Psychophysiology 1968;4:375.
5. Zadra A, Domhoff GW. The content of dreams: methodology and findings. In: Kryger M, Roth T, Dement W, editors. Principles and practices of sleep medicine. 5th edition. Philadelphia: Saunders; 2010. p. 584–95.
6. Domhoff GW. Finding meaning in dreams: a quantitative approach. New York: Plenum; 1996.
7. Hall C. A ubiquitous sex difference in dreams, revisited. J Pers Soc Psychol 1984;46:1109–17.
8. Hall C, Domhoff GW. A ubiquitous sex difference in dreams. J Abnorm Soc Psychol 1963;66:278–80.
9. Schredl M, Petra C, Bishop A, et al. Content analysis of German students' dreams: comparison to American findings. Dreaming 2003;13:237–43.
10. Domhoff GW, Meyer-Gomes K, Schredl M. Dreams as the expression of conceptions and concerns: a comparison of German and American college students. Imagination, Cognition & Personality 2005–6;25:269–82.
11. Foulkes D. Children's dreams. New York: Wiley; 1982.
12. Foulkes D. Children's dreaming and the development of consciousness. Cambridge (MA): Harvard University Press; 1999.
13. Strauch I. Traume im ubergang von der kindheit ins jugendalter: ergebnisse einer langzeitstudie. Bern (Switzerland): Huber; 2004.
14. Strauch I. REM dreaming in the transition from late childhood to adolescence: a longitudinal study. Dreaming 2005;15:155–69.
15. Hall C, Van de Castle R. The content analysis of dreams. New York: Appleton-Century-Crofts; 1966.
16. Domhoff GW, Schneider A. Much ado about very little: the small effect sizes when home and laboratory collected dreams are compared. Dreaming 1999;9:139–51.
17. Hall C. Studies of dreams collected in the laboratory and at home. Santa Cruz (CA): Institute of Dream Research; 1966.
18. Domhoff GW. New directions in the study of dream content using the Hall and Van de Castle coding system. Dreaming 1999;9(2–3):115–37.
19. Hall C. Content analysis of dreams: categories, units, and norms. In: Gerbner G, editor. The analysis of communication content. New York: Wiley; 1969. p. 147–58.
20. Van de Castle R. Problems in applying methodology of content analysis. In: Kramer M, editor. Dream psychology and the new biology of dreaming. Springfield (IL): Charles C. Thomas; 1969. p. 185–97.
21. Domhoff GW. The scientific study of dreams: neural networks, cognitive development, and content analysis. Washington, DC: American Psychological Association; 2003.
22. Cohen J. Statistical power analysis for the behavioral sciences. Mahwah (NJ): Erlbaum; 1988.
23. Domhoff GW, Schneider A. Similarities and differences in dream content at the cross-cultural, gender, and individual levels. Conscious Cogn 2008;17:1257–65.

24. Schneider A, Domhoff GW. DreamBank. Available at: www.dreambank.net. Accessed February 11, 2010.

25. Bulkeley K. Seeking patterns in dream content: a systematic approach to word searches. Conscious Cogn 2009;18:909–16.

26. Domhoff GW, Schneider A. Studying dream content using the archive and search engine on DreamBank.net. Conscious Cogn 2008;17:1238–47.

27. Underwood M. Social aggression among girls. New York: Guilford; 2003.

28. Kramer M. A review of dreaming by psychiatric patients: an update. Santa Cruz (CA): Association for the Study of Dreams; 1999.

29. Kramer M, Roth T. Dreams in psychopathology. In: Wolman B, editor. Handbook of dreams. New York: Van Nostrand Reinhold; 1979. p. 361–7.

30. Hall C. A comparison of the dreams of four groups of hospitalized mental patients with each other and with a normal population. J Nerv Ment Dis 1966; 143:135–9.

31. Schnetzler J, Carbonel B. Etude thématique des recits de rêves de sujets normaux, schizophrènes et autres psychotiques [A thematic study of dream reports for normal subjects, schizophrenics, and other psychotic patients]. Annales Medíco Psychologiques 1976;3:367–80 [in French].

32. Gentil M, Lader M. Dream content and daytime attitudes in anxious and calm women. Psychol Med 1978;8:297–304.

33. Kramer M, Roth T. Comparison of dream content in laboratory dream reports of schizophrenic and depressive patient groups. Compr Psychiatry 1973;14:325–9.

34. Allport G. The use of personal documents in psychological science. New York: Social Science Research Council; 1942.

35. Baldwin A. Personal structure analysis: a statistical method for investigating the single personality. J Abnorm Soc Psychol 1942;37:163–83.

36. Webb E, Campbell D, Schwartz R, et al. Nonreactive measures in the social sciences. 2nd edition. Chicago: Rand McNally; 1981.

37. Bulkeley K. The religious content of dreams: à new scientific foundation. Pastoral Psychol 2009;58:93–106.

38. Hall C, Domhoff GW. The dreams of Freud and Jung. Psychol Today 1968;2:42–5.

39. Hall C, Nordby V. The individual and his dreams. New York: New American Library; 1972.

40. Roussy F. Testing the notion of continuity between waking experience and REM dream content. Dissertation Abstracts International: Section B. 2000; 61(2-B):1106.

41. Roussy F, Brunette M, Mercier P, et al. Daily events and dream content: unsuccessful matching attempts. Dreaming 2000;10(2):77–83.

42. Roussy F, Camirand C, Foulkes D, et al. Does early-night REM dream content reliably reflect presleep state of mind? Dreaming 1996;6:121–30.

43. Bell A, Hall C. The personality of a child molester: an analysis of dreams. Chicago: Aldine; 1971.

44. Domhoff GW. The repetition of dreams and dream elements: a possible clue to a function of dreams. In: Moffitt A, Kramer M, Hoffmann R, editors. The functions of dreams. Albany (NY): State University of New York Press; 1993. p. 293–320.

Sleep States, Memory Processing, and Dreams

Carlyle Smith, PhD

KEYWORDS

• Sleep • Sleep states • Memory • Learning • Dreams

Sleep and memory have historically been studied in isolation from each other. However, in the last 40 years, understanding of the relationship between sleep states and memory processes has made considerable progress. The examination of dream activity as it relates to memory processing during sleep states is in its infancy. Despite this, there are some interesting studies that should form the basis for more research in this area. This paper describes each of the concepts of memory, sleep states, and their relationship, followed by an examination of the nature of dream mentation during postlearning sleep.

MEMORY

Memory, from either a cognitive or neurophysiologic perspective, is not a unitary phenomenon. The term should be used as a generic concept for information storage, and includes several specific subcategories.

There is believed to be a short-term memory that can last from seconds to minutes. At this stage, the newly acquired information is believed to be volatile and unstable. The learned material is then believed to be transformed into a more permanent long-term memory store. The information is believed to be converted into a more permanent stable state that takes place over a period of hours, days, and possibly even years. This dynamic process is referred to as memory consolidation, which can be defined as the time-dependent process that converts labile memory traces into a more permanent form.

There are now understood to be several different memory systems that are relatively independent of each other. One of the models of memory suggests that there are 2 main memory systems, declarative and nondeclarative, that are served by different neural structures.[1]

Declarative material is easily accessible to verbal description, and encoding and retrieval are usually performed explicitly. The subject is consciously aware of the information that is to be learned and aware that it can be accessed when desired from memory store. Declarative memory is further categorized into semantic and episodic components. Semantic memories comprise our factual knowledge of the world. For example, most individuals know that Paris is the capital city of France. However, they probably do not remember when or where they acquired this information. This distinguishes semantic memory from episodic memory. Episodic memories include the information of interest as well as their contextual location in time and space. Being able to recall what you ate for dinner as well as the fine details of where you were and who was with you is an example of an episodic memory.

By contrast, nondeclarative memories are not easily accessible to verbal description. Usually, learning occurs implicitly or without conscious awareness. This means that our behavior can be modified without our conscious awareness. Assessment that nondeclarative memories exist can best be done by observing behavior. If someone says that they have learned how to skate, the best way to be assured that this is so would be to ask the individual to put on a skating demonstration for you.

Within the category of nondeclarative types of learning there are several subtypes. They include procedural memory (the learning of skills and habits), priming, and simple classic conditioning

Department of Psychology, Trent University, 1600 West Bank Drive, Peterborough, Ontario K9J 7B8, Canada
E-mail address: csmith@trentu.ca

Sleep Med Clin 5 (2010) 217–228
doi:10.1016/j.jsmc.2010.01.002
1556-407X/10/$ – see front matter Crown Copyright © 2010 Published by Elsevier Inc. All rights reserved.

(which includes emotional responses and skeletal musculature responses). These learning subtypes are subtended by different neural substrates and are thus considered to be relatively independent learning systems.[1]

SLEEP STATES

The states of sleep are now conventionally divided into 2 separate categories: rapid eye movement (REM) and non–rapid eye movement (NREM) sleep. NREM sleep is further divided into several categories. Sleep onset in humans is characterized by a light stage of sleep (Stage 1) which typically only lasts for a few minutes in healthy young adults. This stage gives way to Stage 2 sleep, a deeper stage of sleep with special features on an electroencephalogram (EEG), including the spindle and K-complex. The most prominent background EEG is theta (5–7 Hz). This stage of sleep is more enduring and comprises about 50% of the sleep night. Deeper and more profound sleep is labeled Stage 3/4 sleep and it is characterized by slow (delta) waves (1–4 Hz). There are no rapid eye movements in NREM and although tension in the large muscle groups is much reduced, it is still present. By contrast, REM sleep is composed of faster EEG frequencies (7–10 Hz) and complete muscle atonia for all of the large muscle groups. Periodic rapid eye movements occur in this sleep state. These movements do not occur in any of the other sleep states.

Throughout the sleep night there is an ultradian rhythm of 90 minutes, which is quite robust. The healthy young adult begins the night with a few minutes of Stage 1, but quickly drops to Stage 2. Stage 2 turns into Stage 3 (with between 20% and 50% delta waves) and then into Stage 4 (with more than 50% delta waves). Stages 3 and 4 are considered to be electrophysiologically similar and are often grouped together as a single stage called slow wave sleep (SWS). After Stage 3/4, the sleep then lightens and Stage 2 is again observed. In the first 90-minute sleep period of the night, Stage 2 is followed by the first episode of REM sleep, which is relatively short (approximately 10 minutes). Thus, at the end of the first sleep cycle, the individual has typically had 80 minutes of NREM sleep and 10 minutes of REM. As the cycles repeat, the time spent in Stages 3/4 declines, whereas the amount of time spent in REM sleep increases. By the last cycle of the night, there is very little Stage 3/4, but the number of minutes of REM sleep has increased, and the final REM period can last 30 minutes or longer; the NREM sleep is composed almost entirely of Stage 2.[2]

SLEEP STATES AND MEMORY CONSOLIDATION

Three main approaches have been used to examine the relationship between sleep and memory processes. (1) One method has been to look at the changes in sleep EEG following task acquisition compared with baseline values. More recently, the added use of brain imaging techniques such as positron emission tomography (PET) and functional magnetic resonance imaging (fMRI) has added to the understanding of post-learning brain changes during sleep. (2) The second approach has been to examine the result of sleep deprivation following learning compared with normal postacquisition sleep. To avoid possible stress confounds, more recent studies have used a day-night design. The control group has a test-retest interval of 12 hours with no intervening sleep (such as 10 AM to 10 PM). The test group also has a 12-hour test-retest interval, but for them, the 12-hour interval includes a night of sleep (such as 10 PM to 10 AM). (3) The third approach has been to use various kinds of sensory stimulation during postlearning sleep to examine the possibility of memory enhancement.

DECLARATIVE MEMORY AND SLEEP

Using these various approaches, it seems clear that sleep states are beneficial for memory consolidation. However, different kinds of sleep are differentially beneficial for certain types of memory over other types. Declarative memory has been studied in its semantic and episodic forms. For episodic memory, a large number of studies have examined the effect of sleep on verbal material such as paired-associate words and prose passages. Explicit encoding of landscapes, object locations, faces or visuospatial memory, and navigation within virtual or natural environments has also been studied. Generally, it has been reported that SWS sleep is most beneficial for these kinds of memories.[3–7] Other studies have concluded that Stage 2 sleep is also important, with most observing an increase in Stage 2 sleep spindle activity.[8–12] Improvement in declarative memory has also been reported, either by directly enhancing SWS activity using direct current[13] or by directly boosting the level of slow oscillations following declarative learning.[14] One study has shown that although the improvements following sleep in explicit recall for word pairs in a paired-associate task is small, the ability to keep multiple lists separate is greatly improved.[15,16] SWS and Stage 2 have been reported to be involved in preliminary work using this retroactive interference paradigm.[17] A smaller number of studies have reported that REM sleep was important for this type of memory. In 1 study, memory of the specific spatial and temporal features of the word pairs was impaired by REM sleep deprivation.[18] In a second study the power of sigma and theta bands was observed to increase at central brain sites during the REM sleep following paired-associate learning.[19]

Fewer studies have looked at the role of sleep in semantic memory. Two studies have combined imaging with EEG to show that acquisition of paired associates[5] or pictures of landscapes[20] began with increased activity in the hippocampus but 6 months later, recall was associated with more activity in the medial prefrontal cortex (mPFC). Although the studies did not assess to what degree the memories had become semanticized, they did show that successful acquisition was positively correlated with the amount of SWS and that the area where memories were stored had changed from the more temporary site of the hippocampus to the more permanent site of the mPFC over a period of months. For the paired-associate study, sleep deprivation resulted in a weaker mPFC activation than a night of regular sleep when assessed 6 months later. This indicates that sleep deprivation leads to long-lasting changes in degree of memory consolidation.[5]

NONDECLARATIVE MEMORY AND SLEEP

Generally implicitly acquired memories may be relatively independent in terms of neural and cognitive substrates.[1] Skills and habits refer to acquisition of novel perceptual, motor, and cognitive abilities with repeated practice (such as perceptual discrimination, skating, and so forth). For example, visual perceptual learning involving a texture discrimination task has shown that REM and SWS should be involved for the most efficient acquisition of this task.[21–25]

For pure motor skill acquisition, such as the well-studied finger-tapping task, it is known that there is postsleep improvement, which seems related to Stage 2 sleep.[26–28] For more complex perceptual motor skills, such as the rotary pursuit task, Stage 2[29–31] and REM[31] sleep have both been implicated. For a more cognitively demanding task such as the mirror-tracing task, REM sleep seemed to be the more important sleep state[3,32,33] although improvement was also seen after non-REM naps.[34] It has been proposed that these discrepancies can be explained by the initial skill levels of the individual participants. In 1 pursuit-rotor study, it was observed that participants with low initial skill levels learned the task and showed corresponding increases in REM sleep. On the other hand, subjects who had high initial skill levels showed increases in Stage 2 sleep variables. It was proposed that individuals were using 1 of 2 overlapping consolidation systems depending on their previous experience. Subjects who found the task required them to come up with a new cognitive strategy showed increases in REM sleep. Those individuals who had some previous experience on the same type of task were simply refining and elaborating existing memories and showed Stage 2 sleep changes. This idea is consistent with REM sleep activity reported following acquisition of more complex perceptual motor[35,36] and cognitive[37–39] tasks. The idea that REM sleep is more important for consolidation of higher-order implicitly learned information is further supported by other studies reporting REM sleep changes.[33,40–42]

EMOTIONAL MEMORY

The role of sleep in consolidation of emotionally charged memories has only recently been examined.[43–49] Generally, emotional memories were better consolidated after periods of REM sleep compared with NREM sleep.[44,49] Emotional memories may be more resistant to total sleep deprivation.[43,46]

Hu and colleagues[45] studied the effects of sleep on memory for neutral and emotionally arousing pictures. They found that if sleep intervened between training and retest, participants showed superior memory for the emotionally arousing pictures. In another study, it was reported that brief sleep after acquisition of emotional text was sufficient to keep those memories alive for 4 years when retesting was done. The neutral material, by contrast, was not well remembered. The investigators suggested that this process might well have relevance for the treatment of posttraumatic sleep disorder victims and proposed the idea that sleep deprivation following an emotional event might alleviate this problem.[50] However, in a brain imaging study (fMRI), participants were either allowed a night of sleep or were sleep deprived. It was observed that positive emotional stimuli were impaired on retest in the sleep-deprived group compared with the rested group, but negative emotional memories were not impaired. Although hippocampal-cortical connections were weaker in the group that had been deprived sleep, they showed an alternate amygdalo-cortical network activity. They concluded that negative and potentially dangerous information was stored by means of an alternative brain network despite sleep deprivation. Such a result suggests that sleep deprivation alone will not allow negative emotional material to be forgotten.

SLEEP-DEPENDENT MECHANISMS OF MEMORY CONSOLIDATION

Ponto-geniculo-occipital (PGO) waves have been extensively studied in animals. They consist of phasic bioelectric potentials, originating in the pons, that are closely related to the rapid eye movements of REM sleep. Increases in this PGO activity have been observed in rats following acquisition of an avoidance task.[51,52] Similar mechanisms are believed to exist in humans.[53–55] Several human studies have reported increases in REM density following procedural learning.[33,40,56]

One study presented sounds in the background while the subject was learning a complex logic task. Maximum memory enhancement was observed when the same sounds (<waking threshold) were again presented during REM sleep to coincide in time with the actual rapid eye movements. Presentations of the sound during tonic REM sleep did not produce any memory increases. Results further reinforce the idea that PGO activity is an important mechanism for efficient brain plasticity.[57]

Hippocampal theta rhythm (4–7 Hz) of the hippocampus is a prominent signature of REM sleep in animals and humans.[58] It is theorized that cortical information activates the hippocampal CA3 system during learning associated with waking and REM sleep theta. During subsequent SWS, previously activated neurons are re-activated during sharp wave bursts. Memory transiently stored in CA3 region can be transferred to cortical regions.[58] Several studies support the idea of hippocampal to cortical transfer.[5,20,59]

Sleep spindles have long been a distinctive characteristic of Stage 2 sleep although they are also observed in SWS to a much lesser extent. The original 12 to 14 Hz spindle-shaped EEG bursts lasting approximately 0.5 to 1.5 seconds have now been expanded to include frequencies of 11.5 to 16.5 Hz.[60] Spindle generation has been considered an ideal mechanism for synaptic plasticity and involves thalamo-cortical connections. Several studies have reported an increase in spindle density following declarative memory task acquisition.[8,9,11,61] Similarly, for procedural memory, Stage 2 spindle increases were observed following acquisition of a simple motor task[27,28,62] and a perceptual motor task.[19,30] As mentioned previously, 1 theory suggests that the spindle may represent a component of 1 memory

processing subsystem that is in use when individuals are already somewhat familiar with the material to be learned.[32]

Slow waves (<4 Hz) may regulate spindle oscillations that are believed to be important for memory consolidation.[63] Brain regional increases in SWS have been observed following motor task acquisition[64] suggesting local homeostatic mechanisms for memory consolidation.[65] Memory enhancement was observed when slow oscillations (<1 Hz) were imposed on participants during postlearning sleep during normal SWS, also suggesting a facility role for slow oscillatory EEG activity.

SUMMARY OF SLEEP AND MEMORY LITERATURE

Different kinds of memory seem to involve different stages of sleep to further the process of memory consolidation. Declarative learning seems to invoke NREM (SWS and/or Stage 2) with less participation for REM sleep. For nondeclarative learning, depending on the type of task, SWS, Stage 2, or REM, or all of these, might be involved. It seems likely that implicit learning requiring new cognitive strategies might involve REM sleep more than NREM sleep. Tasks that are either explicit or for which the participant has had some previous experience seem to favor Stage 2 sleep. Emotionally charged memories favor recruitment of REM sleep processes.

DREAMS AND SLEEP STATES

For the purpose of this article, dreams are defined as mental activity reported on awakening from a sleep state.

Traditionally, dreams were considered to be occurring during REM sleep with very little mentation during other sleep states.[66] More recent work has indicated that dream reports can also be obtained from subjects awakened from the other stages of sleep.[67] Although some investigators have argued that REM- and NREM-derived dreams may not differ qualitatively,[68] awakenings from REM sleep still provide the highest frequency of dream reports.[69,70] Dream mentation from awakenings at sleep onset has been found to yield reports 35% of the time.[69] For NREM sleep, the rate has been reported to range from 43% to 60%[69,70] and for REM awakenings, the percentage of recall was more than 80%.[69,70] REM reports are considered to be longer[68,71] as well as more vivid and bizarre compared with NREM dreams.[72,73]

DREAMS AND MEMORY IN CHILDREN

It is well known that children in the lower age groups have different amounts of the stages of sleep than adults. The basic sleep state architecture patterns observed in adults are also observed in children after about 3 years of age, but the percentages of each sleep stage are different. In children, there are more hours of sleep and the percentage of SWS sleep is higher. The percentage of REM sleep is also higher than in adults. Thus, the sleep system, despite changes with age, is intact and functional from a very young age.[74]

Only a few laboratory studies have examined the relationship between sleep states and memory in young children.[75,76] Sleep aids declarative memory consolidation but not procedural memory consolidation. Thus, the sleep-memory system seems to be active in young children, but may not be mature.

The situation with respect to dreams in the very young, also suggests some immaturity. Young children do not show the high level of dream reporting from REM awakenings seen in adults. In several careful dream collection studies, children less than 9 to 11 years of age showed a median recall rate of 20% to 30%, much lower than the approximate 80% or more seen in adults. Similarly, recall from NREM awakenings was only 6% in the young, but rose to about 40% in young teenagers. Until ages 13 to 15 years, the dream reports had a different content. In the very young, REM dream reports were usually composed of single images that did not move. At ages 5 to 8 years, dream characters moved around, but dream narratives were not well developed, compared with adult dreams. The maturity of dream reports seemed to parallel cognitive maturity and remained relatively immature until the development of good visuospatial skills.[77–79]

It is clear that children are learning many things at these young ages and are undoubtedly using REM and NREM sleep. However, although no dreams have been collected in a sleep-memory experimental situation with young children, it seems unlikely at this point that their dreams are necessary for, or reflect the ongoing consolidation of memories during sleep.

DREAM DELAY: DO RELEVANT DREAMS ALWAYS OCCUR THE NIGHT FOLLOWING TASK ACQUISITION?

Most sleep-memory studies in animals and in humans have looked exclusively at the first few hours of sleep or the first night of sleep following task acquisition to examine the nature of the sleep consolidation mechanisms. However, there are a few studies that have looked at sleep following acquisition for more than a single posttraining day and have found sleep state changes that continue for at least several days after the end of training. In rats, REM sleep increases have been observed to persist for up to a week after the end of avoidance task acquisition.[80,81] Similarly, in humans, increases in REM sleep parameters have been observed 2 to 3 days after the end of the acquisition period.[40,82] Other laboratories have also noted the persistence of sleep-related consolidation several days after training.[83]

There is some evidence of a cyclic recurring dream content and a review has been done by Nielsen.[84] The results of several studies indicate that the events dreamed about on a given day were then not dreamed about for 5 to 7 days, when participants once more dreamed on the same topic as on day 1 (circaseptan rhythms). The dreams identified included self-selection of the most meaningful/significant events in their lives[85] or manipulation of an external stimulus, including the wearing of goggles with red filters[86] or an emotionally upsetting film.[87] It might be imagined that there was a longer-term sleep state adjustment to the red goggles, for example, because it is known that wearing inverted prisms results in REM sleep parameter changes[88] as well as dream incorporation.[89] It is premature to say that dreams are related to long-term post-learning increases. There would not seem to be any human studies that have recorded sleep states for a week after task acquisition and that have awakened their subjects to obtain dream reports under learning conditions. Such experiments might provide a fruitful avenue for future research. One group has reported qualitative differences in memory sources of recent versus delayed (about 1 week) dreams about significant life events,[85] suggesting an ongoing process of memory transfer from 1 brain site to another.

EXAMINATION OF DREAM CONTENT FOLLOWING TASK ACQUISITION

If dreams reflect memory-processing activity, one might expect a correspondence between dreams from a given sleep state and the type of learning taking place. It has been suggested that there is a homology between dream content and memory type. REM dreams, being more hallucinatory, emotional, and bizarre,[72] would be present during emotional memory consolidation, whereas NREM dreams, being more thoughtlike and less hallucinatory,[69] would be involved in more neutral tasks such as memorization of word pairs with REM sleep consolidating emotional memories.[90]

Given the number of tasks that have now been examined and the sleep states implicated in subsequent memory processing, it seems clear that a more precise examination of this idea has yet to be done. For example, whereas REM sleep seems involved with emotional memory consolidation,[44] it is also involved with tasks that require a new cognitive strategy,[33] including simple perceptual motor tasks[91] that are not particularly emotional.

Not many studies have looked at dream content following the task acquisition, and these few have examined REM dreams. In 1 study, the subjects were asked for their dreams after continuously wearing inverted prisms for 4 days. REM dream reports were collected on nights 3 and 4. Although subjects had few direct incorporations of the experience, they did exhibit indirect metaphorical content (eg, "I wanted to know what it was. Then I looked at a word but it was upside down…"). The dreams generally reflected increases in motor and visual difficulties, as well as misfortunes and dreamer confusion.[92]

In another study, this laboratory examined the changes in dream content during prolonged (several weeks) exposure to French language learning. In terms of sleep states, they found that progress in language learning was correlated with increases in the percentage of REM sleep. For dream content, the more learning progress made, the more French incorporations and French communications were observed. In addition, learning progress was significantly correlated with latency to first French language incorporation into a dream. Those individuals who made little or no progress in learning the language did not report any French language incorporations in their dreams. The results of this study suggest that a minimum level of learning must occur before the dream content is affected. There would also seem to be a gradient, by which more learning reflected more French content. At first glance, this task might be considered declarative in type, but it is probably a mix of declarative and procedural, because language learning is much more complex than just word memorization.

Another group has recently reported a correlation between learning progress and REM dream elements after the acquisition of a complex computer game. The number of game-related elements in dreams correlated with performance gains according to an inverted-U function.[93]

Examination of dream content from awakenings just after sleep onset was performed using the Tetris computer game,[94] which participants played for about 2 hours daily for 3 to 4 days. Subjects were novices, experts, and amnesics (temporal lobe damage). All participants saw similar mental images from sleep onset awakenings. The novices reported seeing the puzzle pieces falling; the experts sometimes had the added experience of recognizing the pieces falling as being from their own games, years ago. The pieces were recognizable in terms of color and sound. The amnesics also reported falling pieces, but they were unable to remember having played the game or to recognize the experimenter from session to session. A second study[73,95] used a simulated downhill skiing simulator (Alpine Racer) as the task. Subjects awakened at sleep onset reported visual and kinesthetic sensations of skiing down the hill. Those individuals who had previous skiing experience sometimes reported images from prior skiing experiences. The images usually had high emotional salience, such as places where the subjects tended to crash.

Several interesting conclusions have been drawn from these data. The memories that were retrieved during the sleep onset period were assessed as originating from a semantic memory source rather than from an episodic (hippocampal) source. There were virtually no reports of seeing the room where the experiment was held, the computer itself, the keyboard, or the desk holding the apparatus. In addition, the amnesic subjects were unable to process episodic memories at any time, but could still recall the falling game pieces. This conclusion is consistent with another study that examined the small percentage of home-report dreams recalled that contained actual episodic replay of previous daytime events (1%–2%).[96] It is also consistent with the hypothesis, derived from animal studies, that there is no hippocampal outflow through the entorhinal cortex to the cerebral cortex during REM sleep.[97,98]

For the Tetris game, there was some evidence that this dream imagery was inversely related to task proficiency, for novices and for experts. Lack of imagery seemed to predict better performance. These results were interesting in that they might provide an indicator of the initial skill level of the participant. In sleep-memory studies using the rotary pursuit task, individuals with high initial skill levels showed postsleep changes in Stage 2 sleep architecture, whereas subjects with low initial skill levels showed postlearning sleep changes in REM sleep. These results were consistent with a theory that there are least 2 sleep-memory subsystems, one subserved by Stage 2 sleep and the other by REM sleep mechanisms.[32] Could it be that the best performers (measured by initial Tetris performance) did not direct their memory processing to REM sleep-related mechanisms, but rather to the Stage 2 NREM sleep-memory system? Although the Tetris and Alpine Racer games are more complex than the rotary pursuit task, it seems possible that the participants might choose REM if they found the task novel, requiring a new cognitive strategy, and would choose the Stage 2 system if they already had done similar activities and treated the task as one where mostly refinement was needed and no new cognitive strategy was required. Although the dreams were collected from dream onset, and there is no way of telling whether related dream mental activity might have appeared in either REM or Stage 2 sleep, it seems possible that the memory processing system chosen might already be made at the time of sleep onset imagery.

There was also some evidence that delayed incorporation (subject was allowed 2 hours of sleep before being awakened) resulted in more remote mental imagery, obviously related to the task, but modified. This phenomenon was also reported in delayed sleep mentation from the Alpine Racer task (eg, instead of skiing down the hill, they dreamed of "falling down a hill" or "moving through some kind of forest" with their "entire upper body … incredibly straight"). It was concluded that the more directly related images had been replaced by more weakly associated images.[73,95]

In a study using declarative material, subjects were required to memorize nonsense sentences. Then during subsequent sleep they were awakened from REM sleep to provide dream reports. The content was judged to be related to the previously memorized sentences, although it manifested as words and phrases associated with the original words rather than the words themselves.[99] These results are consistent with the finding that associations made just after awakenings from REM sleep tend to be secondary weaker associations than those made from the waking state. It has been argued that the participants awakened from REM sleep are making their choices with a brain that is still, at least partially, a REM sleep brain.[73,100,101]

In a memory enhancement study,[57] participants were trained in a cognitive procedural task (complex logic task). A clicking sound was present in the background during acquisition and acted as the conditioned stimulus (CS). During the post-learning sleep night, subjects were subjected to these CS clicks via a mini-earphone. The clicks were timed to coincide with the maximum deflection of the rapid eye movements of REM sleep. On retest, the experimental group showed

memory for the task that was significantly better than the control groups, with a 23% enhancement. The click cues were believed to have acted as reminders for the participants to remember to process the task. In a second related study,[102] subjects were presented with a REM-dependent[33] cognitive procedural task (mirror trace) accompanied by the background CS clicks. The task required subjects to try and draw a pencil line inside the margins of complex figures by looking in a mirror. They were then given subthreshold postacquisition CS clicks during REM sleep as before. However, they were then awakened after an estimated 50% to 80% of the REM period was over to obtain a dream report. Compared with control groups, the dream narratives of the test group were significantly longer. The groups did not differ on time spent in any sleep stage including REM sleep. Thus it is possible that the dreams of the test group were somehow more intense. There seemed to be many detailed references to cars and driving and so a detailed lexicon was developed and used to score the dreams in content analysis fashion, taking care to control for dream length. The test group showed significantly more references to cars, driving, driving problems and so forth. Thus, the most popular metaphor for keeping the pencil between the lines of the figures they traced in the mirror seemed to be about cars and driving. No one reported episodic types of dreams such as "trying to draw a figure while looking in a mirror," supporting other research which has found very little episodic memory replay.[96]

The results are consistent with the idea that individuals use dream themes of previous experiences that are familiar to them to characterize more novel present problems.[95,103] In this experiment, they related the problem of trying to keep a pencil on track to a dream of trying to keep a vehicle on the road. The mental representations were of a negative nature, even though learning occurred (eg, "… he started driving down the street and … he cut through a neighborhood and was going really fast and crashed into a house"). There were no positive or success dreams of being able to avoid driving mistakes and mishaps. These increases in negative outcomes and misfortunes were also reported by subjects adapting to the inverted prisms.[92]

NEURAL STRUCTURES INVOLVED IN DREAM GENERATION

The original activation-synthesis hypothesis[104] suggested that dreams are produced primarily during REM sleep by mechanisms in the pons that randomly bombard the visual cortex during REM sleep. More recent theory revisions include the possibility of REM intrusions into NREM sleep states and a more complete description of the mental states against the background of transmitter modulation. There is a strong emphasis on the role of the cholinergic transmitter system during REM dream generation. In addition, it is assumed that there is a complex forebrain network that plays a major role in shaping dream content.[72] Stickgold[73] has proposed an error detection model of dream construction, based on the error detection model of Cohen.[105] In this model, the brain is presumed to evaluate the potential value of novel forms of behavior during REM sleep. Weak cortical associations are preferentially activated during REM,[100] in the absence of dorsolateral prefrontal cortical (DLPFC) input or hippocampal feedback.[97] There is an active error detection system originating in the anterior cingulated cortex and including emotional evaluation by the amygdala and medial orbitofrontal cortex. All of the aforementioned theories are based on the original ideas of the activation-synthesis hypothesis, although many structures have now been added.

An alternative to models based on activation-synthesis comes from the work of Solms.[106] His neuropsychological information was obtained from patients with brain lesions and suggested that several other brain structures are important for normal dream activity. Damage to medial prefrontal or parieto-temporal-occipital junction areas resulted in dream deficits, whereas lesions of the temporal lobes resulted in an increase in nightmares. Increased intensity of dreaming involved damage to medial prefrontal, anterior cingulate, or basal forebrain areas. The model de-emphasizes the role of the brainstem in dream generation. Although sufficient brain activation is deemed necessary, it is argued that the dream generation transmitter system is dopaminergic and originates in the ventral tegmentum, just above the pons. This system fans out to the amygdala, the anterior cingulate gyrus, and frontal cortex. A detailed critique of these theories can be found in Domhoff.[107]

Despite some theoretic differences, it seems clear that the DLPFC is not active and that there is no hippocampus-to-cortex information flow during REM sleep. This is believed to account for the lack of attention to unusual incongruities that occur in the dream. An advantage might be that the weaker (but novel) associations made would result in creative new ways of solving problems. It has been reported that solutions to a novel math problem were solved much more quickly by students following a night of sleep compared with an equal time awake.[108] Unfortunately, no dreams were collected in this study. According to the error detection model, the evaluation of the novel associations would be evaluated by the amygdala and orbitofrontal cortex in the presence of the anterior cingulate cortex. The dream would be generated based on the relative activities of these brain structures.[95]

SOME GENERAL CONCLUSIONS

Despite the meager data available at present to decide the relationship of the memory consolidation process during sleep and dream mentation, some tentative conclusions can be made. It is likely that dream generation is not episodic in nature and that the images generated use semantic memories that are somehow linked together. It would explain why learning new information often gives rise to dream images of related material. Very little sleep-memory work has been directed at this kind of memory.

The dreams of children are very primitive although many things that they learn are quite complex and sophisticated, which suggests that dreams are not absolutely necessary for sleep-related memory consolidation.

The fact that task experts produced relevant dream images of an earlier time in their lives (eg, the Tetris experiment) suggests that dreams are at least reflecting a cataloguing process for storing similar experiences together (if we can assume sleep onset and later dream activity are part of the same dream-generating process).[73]

Dreams with negative outcomes do not necessarily mean lack of learning progress. This mental activity may simply be a read-out of the ongoing process.

Gauging learning progress from dreams later in the night was positively correlated with the French immersion study, but appeared to be inversely correlated in the Tetris and Alpine motor skill studies. A critical factor may be the initial level of proficiency of a participant. One explanation, as previously mentioned, is that the subjects who found the task to be generally familiar used a memory consolidation system associated with Stage 2 sleep. It is possible that the mental activity associated with this system is different from that of the less proficient subjects who needed a new cognitive strategy and were thus invoking the REM sleep system.

It would seem that dream mentation does reflect recent learning, although it would not seem to be necessary. In some complex tasks, mentation might be helpful in creating new ways of looking at a problem.

FUTURE DIRECTIONS

It seems clear that there is differential involvement of different sleep states in the various types of memory tasks. However, the few studies done have only examined REM dreams and sleep onset mental activity. We have no idea if tasks that use subsequent Stage 2 sleep, such as a perceptual motor task, would provide dreams during this stage reflective of the task being learned. Would the REM dreams from the same task also show this activity or would they be reflective of other problems of a more cognitive or emotional nature? Similarly would a task that is known to involve REM sleep provide similar dream content from REM and NREM dream awakenings? There is some information that REM dreams through the night have a similar theme and seem to be related to ongoing life problems.[109] However, there do not seem to be any instances of a learning situation where REM and NREM dreams were collected. Studies following task acquisition that would examine dreams from awakenings through the night in NREM and REM sleep would be invaluable in tracing the dream changes in parallel with memory-processing activity.

To find the answer to the question of whether dreams are related to memory processing, care must be taken to use objective techniques for collecting and scoring the dreams. One author notes that subjects should receive direction in how to recall dreams (self-observation) so that crucial information is not lost.[110] The content analysis methodology has provided a systematic way of scoring dreams that is reliable and has acceptable statistical procedures.[107] Although it can sometimes not be specific enough for the elements of a particular study, it does provide a general method that can be followed to ensure that dream elements are uniformly scored and reliably compared.

Virtually all of the studies on sleep and memory have assumed that the most important night is the first night after training. However, there are a substantial number of studies that suggest memory processing persists for days and weeks after the end of acquisition. Dream activity at these times has yet to be examined.

Dreaming in children seems to be immature for the early years of life. Yet children obviously learn at a rapid pace. Developmental studies aimed at finding when mature dreams become associated with recently learned material have yet to be done.

The study of the change in dream characteristics following learning may well help us to understand the processes whereby dreams are generated. An examination of the dream mentation induced by a specific learning event may help us to gauge learning progress. A within-subject design comparing dream content before and after task acquisition, and using EEG and brain imaging techniques, would provide valuable insights.

REFERENCES

1. Squire LR. Memory systems of the brain: a brief history and current perspective. Neurobiol Learn Mem 2004;82(3):171–7.
2. Carskadon M, Dement W. Normal human sleep: an overview. In: Kryger M, Roth T, Dement W, editors. Principles and practice of sleep medicine. 4th edition. Philadelphia: Elsevier; 2005. p. 13–23.
3. Plihal W, Born J. Effects of early and late nocturnal sleep on declarative and procedural memory. J Cogn Neurosci 1997;9(4):534–47.
4. Plihal W, Born J. Effects of early and late nocturnal sleep on priming and spatial memory. Psychophysiology 1999;36(5):571–82.
5. Gais S, Albouy G, Boly M, et al. Sleep transforms the cerebral trace of declarative memories. Proc Natl Acad Sci U S A 2007;104(47):18778–83.
6. Tucker MA, Hirota Y, Wamsley EJ, et al. A daytime nap containing solely non-REM sleep enhances declarative but not procedural memory. Neurobiol Learn Mem 2006;86(2):241–7.
7. Gais S, Born J. Low acetylcholine during slow-wave sleep is critical for declarative memory consolidation. Proc Natl Acad Sci U S A 2004;101(7):2140–4.
8. Gais S, Molle M, Helms K, et al. Learning-dependent increases in sleep spindle density. J Neurosci 2002;22(15):6830–4.
9. Schmidt C, Peigneux P, Muto V, et al. Encoding difficulty promotes postlearning changes in sleep spindle activity during napping. J Neurosci 2006; 26(35):8976–82.
10. Clemens Z, Fabo D, Halasz P. Twenty-four hours retention of visuospatial memory correlates with the number of parietal sleep spindles. Neurosci Lett 2006;403(1–2):52–6.
11. Clemens Z, Fabo D, Halasz P. Overnight verbal memory retention correlates with the number of sleep spindles. Neuroscience 2005;132(2):529–35.
12. Schabus M, Gruber G, Parapatics S, et al. Sleep spindles and their significance for declarative memory consolidation. Sleep 2004;27(8):1479–85.
13. Marshall L, Molle M, Hallschmid M, et al. Transcranial direct current stimulation during sleep improves declarative memory. J Neurosci 2004; 24(44):9985–92.
14. Marshall L, Helgadottir H, Molle M, et al. Boosting slow oscillations during sleep potentiates memory. Nature 2006;444(7119):610–3.

15. Ellenbogen JM, Hu PT, Payne JD, et al. Human relational memory requires time and sleep. Proc Natl Acad Sci U S A 2007;104(18):7723–8.

16. Ellenbogen JM, Hulbert JC, Stickgold R, et al. Interfering with theories of sleep and memory: sleep, declarative memory, and associative interference. Curr Biol 2006;16(13):1290–4.

17. Smith C, Moran CR, McGilvray MP, et al. Decreases in stage 2 sleep, spindles and sigma power following acquisition of a declarative task. J Sleep Res 2008;17(Suppl 1):270.

18. Rauchs G, Bertran F, Guillery-Girard B, et al. Consolidation of strictly episodic memories mainly requires rapid eye movement sleep. Sleep 2004; 27(3):395–401.

19. Fogel SM, Smith CT, Cote KA. Dissociable learning-dependent changes in REM and non-REM sleep in declarative and procedural memory systems. Behav Brain Res 2007;180(1):48–61.

20. Takashima A, Petersson KM, Rutters F, et al. Declarative memory consolidation in humans: a prospective functional magnetic resonance imaging study. Proc Natl Acad Sci U S A 2006; 103(3):756–61.

21. Gais S, Plihal W, Wagner U, et al. Early sleep triggers memory for early visual discrimination skills. Nat Neurosci 2000;3(12):1335–9.

22. Karni A, Sagi D. Where practice makes perfect in texture discrimination: evidence for primary visual cortex plasticity. Proc Natl Acad Sci U S A 1991; 88(11):4966–70.

23. Stickgold R, Whidbee D, Schirmer B, et al. Visual discrimination task improvement: a multi-step process occurring during sleep. J Cogn Neurosci 2000;12(2):246–54.

24. Mednick S, Nakayama K, Stickgold R. Sleep-dependent learning: a nap is as good as a night. Nat Neurosci 2003;6(7):697–8.

25. Mednick SC, Nakayama K, Cantero JL, et al. The restorative effect of naps on perceptual deterioration. Nat Neurosci 2002;5(7):677–81.

26. Nishida M, Walker MP. Daytime naps, motor memory consolidation and regionally specific sleep spindles. PLoS One 2007;2(4):e341.

27. Morin A, Doyon J, Dostie V, et al. Motor sequence learning increases sleep spindles and fast frequencies in post-training sleep. Sleep 2008;31(8): 1149–56.

28. Walker MP, Brakefield T, Morgan A, et al. Practice with sleep makes perfect: sleep-dependent motor skill learning. Neuron 2002;35(1):205–11.

29. Smith C, MacNeill C. Impaired motor memory for a pursuit rotor task following Stage 2 sleep loss in college students. J Sleep Res 1994;3(4):206–13.

30. Fogel SM, Smith CT. Learning-dependent changes in sleep spindles and stage 2 sleep. J Sleep Res 2006;15(3):250–5.

31. Peters KR, Smith V, Smith CT. Changes in sleep architecture following motor learning depend on initial skill level. J Cogn Neurosci 2007;19(5):817–29.

32. Smith C, Aubrey J, Peters K. Different roles for REM and stage 2 sleep in motor learning: a proposed model. Psychol Belg 2004;44:81–104.

33. Smith CT, Nixon MR, Nader RS. Posttraining increases in REM sleep intensity implicate REM sleep in memory processing and provide a biological marker of learning potential. Learn Mem 2004; 11(6):714–9.

34. Backhaus J, Junghanns K. Daytime naps improve procedural motor memory. Sleep Med 2006;7(6): 508–12.

35. Buchegger J, Fritsch R, Meier-Koll A, et al. Does trampolining and anaerobic physical fitness affect sleep? Percept Mot Skills 1991;73(1):243–52.

36. Buchegger J, Meier-Koll A. Motor learning and ultradian sleep cycle: an electroencephalographic study of trampoliners. Percept Mot Skills 1988; 67(2):635–45.

37. Maquet P. Functional neuroimaging of normal human sleep by positron emission tomography. J Sleep Res 2000;9(3):207–31.

38. Peigneux P, Laureys S, Fuchs S, et al. Learned material content and acquisition level modulate cerebral reactivation during posttraining rapid-eye-movements sleep. Neuroimage 2003;20(1):125–34.

39. Laureys S, Peigneux P, Phillips C, et al. Experience-dependent changes in cerebral functional connectivity during human rapid eye movement sleep. Neuroscience 2001;105(3):521–5.

40. Smith C, Smith D. Ingestion of ethanol just prior to sleep onset impairs memory for procedural but not declarative tasks. Sleep 2003;26(2):185–91.

41. Cajochen C, Knoblauch V, Wirz-Justice A, et al. Circadian modulation of sequence learning under high and low sleep pressure conditions. Behav Brain Res 2004;151(1–2):167–76.

42. De Koninck J, Lorrain D, Christ G, et al. Intensive language learning and increases in rapid eye movement sleep: evidence of a performance factor. Int J Psychophysiol 1989;8(1):43–7.

43. Wagner U, Degirmenci M, Drosopoulos S, et al. Effects of cortisol suppression on sleep-associated consolidation of neutral and emotional memory. Biol Psychiatry 2005;58(11):885–93.

44. Wagner U, Gais S, Born J. Emotional memory formation is enhanced across sleep intervals with high amounts of rapid eye movement sleep. Learn Mem 2001;8(2):112–9.

45. Hu P, Stylos-Allan M, Walker MP. Sleep facilitates consolidation of emotional declarative memory. Psychol Sci 2006;17(10):891–8.

46. Sterpenich V, Albouy G, Boly M, et al. Sleep-related hippocampo-cortical interplay during emotional memory recollection. PLoS Biol 2007;5(11):e282.

47. Atienza M, Cantero JL. Modulatory effects of emotion and sleep on recollection and familiarity. J Sleep Res 2008;17(3):285–94.

48. Payne JD, Stickgold R, Swanberg K, et al. Sleep preferentially enhances memory for emotional components of scenes. Psychol Sci 2008;19(8):781–8.

49. Wagner U, Hallschmid M, Verleger R, et al. Signs of REM sleep dependent enhancement of implicit face memory: a repetition priming study. Biol Psychol 2003;62(3):197–210.

50. Wagner U, Hallschmid M, Rasch B, et al. Brief sleep after learning keeps emotional memories alive for years. Biol Psychiatry 2006;60(7):788–90.

51. Datta S. Avoidance task training potentiates phasic pontine-wave density in the rat: a mechanism for sleep-dependent plasticity. J Neurosci 2000;20:8607–13.

52. Datta S, Li G, Auerbach S. Activation of phasic pontine-wave generator in the rat: a mechanism for expression of plasticity-related genes and proteins in the dorsal hippocampus and amygdala. Eur J Neurosci 2008;27:1876–92.

53. Salzarulo P, Lairy GC, Bancaud J, et al. direct depth recording of the striate cortex during REM sleep in man: are there PGO potentials? Electroencephalogr Clin Neurophysiol 1975;38:199–202.

54. Peigneux P, Laureys S, Fuchs S, et al. Generation of rapid eye movements during paradoxical sleep in humans. Neuroimage 2001;14(3):701–8.

55. Wehrle R, Czisch M, Kaufmann C, et al. Rapid eye movement-related brain activation in human sleep: a functional magnetic resonance imaging study. Neuroreport 2005;16(8):853–7.

56. Mandai O, Guerrien A, Sockeel P, et al. REM sleep modifications following a Morse code learning session in humans. Physiol Behav 1989;46(4):639–42.

57. Smith C, Weeden K. Post training REMs coincident auditory stimulation enhances memory in humans. Psychiatr J Univ Ott 1990;15(2):85–90.

58. Buzsaki G. Theta oscillations in the hippocampus. Neuron 2002;33(3):325–40.

59. Poe GR, Nitz DA, McNaughton BL, et al. Experience-dependent phase-reversal of hippocampal neuron firing during REM sleep. Brain Res 2000;855(1):176–80.

60. De Gennaro L, Ferrara M. Sleep spindles: an overview. Sleep Med Rev 2003;7:423–40.

61. Schabus M, Hoedlmoser K, Pecherstorfer T, et al. Interindividual sleep spindle differences and their relation to learning-related enhancements. Brain Res 2008;1191:127–35.

62. Walker MP, Brakefield T, Allan Hobson J, et al. Dissociable stages of human memory consolidation and reconsolidation. Nature 2003;425(6958):616–20.

63. Molle M, Marshall L, Gais S, et al. Grouping of spindle activity during slow oscillations in human non-rapid eye movement sleep. J Neurosci 2002;22(24):10941–7.

64. Huber R, Ghilardi MF, Massimini M, et al. Local sleep and learning. Nature 2004;430(6995):78–81.

65. Tononi G, Cirelli C. Sleep function and synaptic homeostasis. Sleep Med Rev 2006;10(1):49–62.

66. Dement W, Kleitman N. The relation of eye movements during sleep to dream activity: an objective method for the study of dreaming. J Exp Psychol 1957;53:339–46.

67. Foulkes D. Dream reports from different stages of sleep. J Abnorm Soc Psychol 1962;65:14–25.

68. Antrobus JS. REM and NREM sleep reports: comparison of word frequencies by cognitive classes. Psychophysiology 1983;1983:562–8.

69. Fosse M, Stickgold R, Hobson A. Brain-mind states: reciprocal variation in thoughts and hallucinations. Psychol Sci 2001;12:30–6.

70. Nielsen TA. Mentation in REM and NREM sleep: a review and possible reconciliation of two models. Behav Brain Sci 2000;23:851–66.

71. Stickgold R, Pace-Schott E, Hobson JA. A new paradigm for dream research: mentation reports following spontaneous arousal from REM and NREM sleep recorded in a home setting. Conscious Cogn 1994;3:16–29.

72. Hobson JA, Pace-Schott EF, Stickgold R. Dreaming and the brain: toward a cognitive neuroscience of conscious states. Behav Brain Sci 2000;23:793–842.

73. Stickgold R. Why we dream. In: Kryger M, Roth T, Dement W, editors. Principles and practice of sleep medicine. 4th edition. Philadelphia: Saunders; 2005. p. 579–87.

74. Ohayon MM, Carskadon M, Guilleminault C, et al. Meta-analysis of quantitative sleep parameters from childhood to old age in healthy individuals: developing normative sleep values across the human lifespan. Sleep 2004;27:1255–73.

75. Backhaus J, Hoecksesfeld R, Born J, et al. Immediate as well as delayed post learning sleep but not wakefulness enhances declarative memory consolidation in children. Neurobiol Learn Mem 2008;89:76–80.

76. Wilhelm I, Diekelmann S, Born J. Sleep in children improves memory performance on declarative but not procedural tasks. Learn Mem 2008;15:373–7.

77. Foulkes D. Children's dreams. New York: Wiley; 1982.

78. Foulkes D. Children's dreaming and the development of consciousness. Cambridge (MA): Harvard University Press; 1999.

79. Foulkes D, Hollifield M, Sullivan B, et al. REM dreaming and cognitive skills at ages 5–8: a

cross-sectional study. Int J Behav Dev 1990;13(4): 447–65.

80. Smith C, Lapp L. Prolonged increases in both PS and number of REMS following a shuttle avoidance task. Physiol Behav 1986;36:1053–7.

81. Smith CT. The REM sleep window and memory processing. In: Maquet P, Smith C, Stickgold R, editors. Sleep and brain plasticity. Oxford: Oxford Press; 2003.

82. Smith C, Lapp L. Increases in number of REMs and REM density in humans following an intensive learning period. Sleep 1991;14:325–30.

83. Stickgold R, LaTanya J, Hobson JA. Visual discrimination learning requires sleep after training. Nat Neurosci 2000;3:1237–8.

84. Nielsen T. Chronobiology of dreaming. Philadelphia: Saunders; 2005.

85. Nielsen T, Kuiken D, Alain G, et al. Immediate and delayed incorporation of events into dreams: further replication and implications for dream function. J Sleep Res 2004;13:327–36.

86. Roffwarg H, Herman JH, Bowe-Anders C, et al. The effects of sustained alterations of waking visual input on dream content. In: Arkin A, Antrobus J, Ellman S, editors. The mind in sleep. Hillsdale (NJ): Erlbaum; 1978. p. 295–349.

87. Nielsen T, Powell DA, Cheung JS. Temporal delays in incorporation of events into dreams. Percept Mot Skills 1995;81:95–104.

88. De Koninck J, Prevost F. Le sommeil paradoxal et le traitement de l'information: une exploration par l'inversion du champ visuel [Paradoxical sleep and information processing: a study involving inversion of the visual field]. Can J Psychol 1991; 45(2):125–39 [in French].

89. De Koninck J, Prevost F, Lortie-Lussier M. Vertical inversion of the visual field and REM sleep mentation. J Sleep Res 1996;5:16–20.

90. Stickgold R. Sleep-dependent memory consolidation. Nature 2005;437(7063):1272–8.

91. Peters KR, Smith V, Smith CT. The effect of initial skill level on the relationship between Stage 2 sleep spindles, rapid eye movements and motor learning. J Cogn Neurosci 2006;19:817–29.

92. De Koninck J. Waking experiences and dreams. In: Kryger M, Roth T, Dement W, editors. Principles and practice of sleep medicine. 3rd edition. Philadelphia: Saunders; 2000.

93. Pantoja AL, Faber J, Rocha LH, et al. Assessment of the adaptive value of dreams. Sleep 2009;32:A421.

94. Stickgold R, Malia A, Maguire D, et al. Replaying the game: hypnagogic images in normals and amnesics. Science 2000;290(5490):350–3.

95. Stickgold R. Memory, cognition, and dreams. In: Maquet P, Smith C, Stickgold R, editors. Sleep and brain plasticity. Oxford: Oxford Press; 2003. p. 17–39.

96. Fosse M, Fosse R, Hobson A, et al. Dreaming and episodic memory: a functional dissociation? J Cogn Neurosci 2003;15:1–9.

97. Chrobak JJ, Buzsaki G. Selective activation of deep layer (V-VI) retrohippocampal cortical neurons during hippocampal sharp waves in the behaving rat. J Neurosci 1994;14(10):6160–70.

98. Chrobak JJ, Buzsaki G. High frequency oscillations in the output networks of the hippocampal - entorhinal axis of the freely behaving rat. J Neurosci 1996;16:3056–66.

99. Cipolli C, Bolzani R, Tuozzi G, et al. Active processing of declarative knowledge during REM sleep dreaming. J Sleep Res 2001;10:277–84.

100. Stickgold R, Scott L, Rittenhouse C, et al. Sleep-induced changes in associative memory. J Cogn Neurosci 1999;11(2):182–93.

101. Dinges DF. Are you awake? Cognitive performance and reverie during the hypnopompic state. In: Bootzin RR, Kihlstrom J, Schacter DL, editors. Sleep and cognition. Washington, DC: American Psychological Association; 1990. p. 159–78.

102. Smith C, Hanke J. Memory processing reflected in dreams from rapid eye movement sleep. Sleep 2004;27:A60.

103. Koukkou M, Lehmann D. Dreaming: the functional state shift hypothesis. Br J Psychiatry 1983;142: 221–31.

104. Hobson JA, Stickgold R. The conscious state paradigm: a neurocognitive approach to waking, sleeping, and dreaming. In: Gazzaniga M, editor. The cognitive neurosciences. Cambridge (MA): M.I.T. Press; 1994. p. 1373–89.

105. Cohen JD, Botvinick M, Carter CS. Anterior cingulate and prefrontal cortex: who's in control? Nat Neurosci 2000;3:421–3.

106. Solms M. The neuropsychology of dreams: a clinicoanatomical study. Mahwah (NJ): Lawrence Erlbaum; 1997.

107. Domhoff GW. The scientific study of dreams: neural networks, cognitive development and content analysis. Washington: American Psychological Association; 2003.

108. Wagner U, Gais S, Haider H, et al. Sleep inspires insight. Nature 2004;427:352–5.

109. Cartwright R. Dreams and adaption to divorce. In: Barrett D, editor. Trauma and dreams. Cambridge (MA): Harvard University Press; 1996. p. 179–85.

110. Nielsen TA, Stenstrom P. What are the memory sources of dreaming? Nature 2005;437:1286–9.

Disturbed Dreaming and Emotion Dysregulation

Ross Levin, PhD[a],*, Gary Fireman, PhD[b], Tore Nielsen, PhD[c,d]

KEYWORDS

- Disturbed dreaming • Emotion dysregulation
- AMPHAC/AND model • REM sleep

Perhaps because of their highly emotive nature and often memorable visual imagery, dreams have long been linked to our innermost emotional functioning, ideas that go back to the earliest use of dreams (as in the Bible) as well as Freud[1,2] and Jung's[3] original psychoanalytic conceptualizations of the human mind. More recently, work by such investigators as Maquet and colleagues[4,5] and Hobson and colleagues[6] have demonstrated an isomorphism between the neurophysiologic components of rapid eye movement (REM) sleep (muscle atonia, heightened limbic activation, particularly in the amygdala, the threat detection control center of the brain, deactivation of the prefrontal dorsolateral cortex, and the reciprocal activation of the amenergic and cholinergic systems) with the phenomenal qualities of dreaming (paralysis, heightened expressed emotion, the absence of metacognition and state-dependent amnesia for the dream on awakening). Thus, the neural qualities of REM sleep seem to be particularly suited for the activation of emotionally charged memorial components that may offer clues into a possible function.

Previous work by Kramer[7] and Cartwright[8,9] has long assigned a mood-regulatory function to dreaming. A review of this work is beyond the scope of the present paper, but Kramer and Cartwright have proposed that dreaming serves a type of emotional thermostat that serves to regulate inner well-being. In a series of studies, Kramer (reviewed in Ref.[7]) demonstrated clear markers of emotion shift from evening to morning that was mediated by dream variables. For example, Kramer demonstrated that the absence of dream characters in the last REM dream of the night was the strongest predictor of a downshift of mood from evening to morning. This finding is consistent with the observation that morning mood is often the worst time for individuals with depression and the findings that depressed individuals have more total REM time and significantly shorter REM latency than individuals without depression or the same individuals after remission of symptoms.[10]

Closely related but independent work by Cartwright and colleagues[8,9,11] with samples of women undergoing midlife divorce and marital separation with and without accompanying depression has shown that the level of intensity of dysphoric mood in their dreams as well as dreaming of the ex-spouse reliably predicted waking depression but that the presence of these variables also predicted enhanced recovery on follow up 1 year after divorce, suggesting that the dreams were integral in processing these negative emotions.

Another area of promising work along these lines pertains to the small literature on recurrent dreaming, loosely defined as dreams with a high degree of replicative content. Some studies in this area[12–14] suggest that the active presence of

The first articulation of the AMPHAC/AND model of disturbed dreaming was presented by Levin & Nielsen (2007) in *Psychological Bulletin* and Nielsen & Levin (2007) in *Sleep Medicine Reviews*.

[a] 25 West 86th Street, Suite #3, New York, NY 10024, USA
[b] Department of Psychology, Suffolk University, Boston, MA, USA
[c] Department of Psychiatry, University of Montreal, Montreal, Canada
[d] Dream and Nightmare Lab, Sacre-Coeur Hospital, Montreal, Canada
* Corresponding author.
E-mail address: rosslevin@drrosslevin.com

Sleep Med Clin 5 (2010) 229–239
doi:10.1016/j.jsmc.2010.01.006

recurrent dreams (roughly defined as dreaming the same dream over and over again) connotes a psychological/emotional obstacle that is associated concomitantly with poorer daytime functioning. Once recurrent dreams end, improved waking psychological functioning is often noted.[12]

One obvious limitation to this work is the inability to disentangle the effects of dreaming from their neurophysiologic background, namely REM sleep, the sleep stage most highly associated with dreaming. There is mounting evidence that healthy sleep is integral to healthy emotional functioning and that waking states marked by mood disturbances of emotional dysregulation are often accompanied by and causally preceded by poor sleep.[15–18] In addition, it seems that intact sleep is crucial to the encoding and consolidation of intact memories (eg, Ref.[19]). This is important given the intimate connection between memory and affect regulation, particularly for such clinical disorders as posttraumatic stress disorder (PTSD) and depression.

The present paper focuses on another type of dreaming often implicated in emotion functioning, namely disturbed dreaming (DD), and a recently formulated model of the pathogenesis of these dreams specifically and all dreaming more generally is reviewed (see Refs.[20–23] for more comprehensive discussion of the model). A primary assumption of this model is that dreams have an adaptive function independent from REM sleep (although closely entrained to REM): the reduction or even extinction of fear memories. DDs, vivid dreams often marked by intense dysphoric emotion (predominantly fear but also including rage, guilt, and grief), represent a dysfunction of this regulatory process and are often engendered by high levels of waking stress. For our purposes, the domain of DD includes the broad spectrum of dysphoric dreaming ranging from dreams that are remembered only on awakening (bad dreams) to dreams that result in a nocturnal awakening (nightmares). Although occasional DDs are nearly ubiquitous in the general population,[24] high DD incidence rates (usually defined as weekly episodes) are strongly associated with poorer waking psychological well-being. In addition, DDs (recurrent nightmares in particular) are a defining symptom of PTSD.[20] The authors thus consider all forms of disturbed dreaming to be observable variants of a common underlying process, namely dysphoric imagery produced during sleep, and that the consequences of these variants are largely dictated by waking responses to the imagery (eg, distress).

Perhaps the most robust finding in the DD literature is the strong association between DD frequency and waking psychopathology.[20,21,23,25–31] Because most of these clinical disorders are marked by considerable waking emotional distress, their association with DD suggests that these dreams are related to a personality style characterized by intense reactive emotional distress.[20,23,26,28,32,33] Furthermore, DDs are often precipitated by stressful life events[25,27,34] and there is a strong link between trauma exposure and subsequent DD.[35,36]

A naturalistic study by Wood and colleagues,[37] clearly showed the relation between heightened life stress and increased DD production. They found the incidence of DD to be twice as high immediately after the 1989 San Francisco earthquake in 2 groups in the San Francisco Bay area than in a sample from Arizona, despite equal baseline frequencies. These differences were dose-response specific to proximity to the earthquake epicenter; those who lived closer to the epicenter reported more nightmares.

THE AMPHAC/AND MODEL OF DD GENERATION

Despite a recent proliferation of experimental work on DDs, their pathogenesis has remained largely unexplained. A recently proposed model incorporating advances in cognitive neuroscience, sleep neurophysiology, and fear conditioning, particularly in relation to PTSD and sociocognitive-based diathesis (ie, vulnerability) stress models of psychopathology, supports a multilevel model of dream function and DD production that unites neural and cognitive processes in waking and sleeping.[20,21,23,29,38] The neurophysiologic branch of this model is termed the AMPHAC network, after its presumed underlying neurophysiologic centers: the amygdala (A), the medial prefrontal cortex (MP), the hippocampus (H), and the anterior cingulated cortex (AC). The cognitive branch is termed the Affect Network Dysfunction (AND) model. Together, the 2 branches integrate explanatory concepts at a neural level (ie, a cohesive and interconnected network of limbic and forebrain centers underlying emotional expression and representation) and a cognitive level (ie, a dream production system that transforms fear memories into dream and nightmare imagery) to account for a variety of features associated with nightmare imagery (lack of emotional control, bizarre features, or replay of traumatic memories).

The AMPHAC/AND model stipulates that DD results from dysfunction in a network of affective processes that, during normal dreaming, are presumed to serve the adaptive function of fear memory regulation and extinction. The underlying neurophysiology and biochemistry of REM sleep seems to be primed to activate these systems.[4,6] At the cognitive level, dreaming is proposed to facilitate fear memory extinction by 3 processes: memory element activation, memory element reactivation, and emotional expression. These processes are discussed in greater depth in the following sections.

Memory Element Activation

The first set of processes refers to the increased availability during dreaming of a wide range of memory elements. Memory elements, rather than complete memories, are emphasized, as complete episodic memories do not typically appear during dreaming.[39] Dreaming tends to express memory elements as though original memories had been reduced to more basic units.[40,41] Often, these appear as isolated features, such as an attribute of a familiar place or character. In other instances, several elements may appear together by virtue of their origin in a single past event or their grouping by some other form of organization, such as a script, or a semantic or phonological category. Although memory elements tend to obscure the relation of dreaming to daily experiences, the link is demonstrable by clinical and experimental observation. Clinically, Hartmann[42] has demonstrated that dreams often portray elements of a person's main emotional concerns (eg, stress, trauma) even if visual or auditory details of a specific memory are absent. Experimentally, memory elements have been detected as the day-residues of previous-day experiences.[43–45] Further, these residues may be temporally delayed by up to a week.[40,46] It remains unknown why normal dreaming disproportionately favors the partial activation of memory elements. One possibility is that it reflects a more general organizing principle of memory. For instance, declarative memories may be stored as multiple traces in which bits and pieces of a single experience are saved by structurally distinct memory systems.[47] In the waking state, episodic memories are then reconstituted when needed from the elements stored in these different systems.[48] In the dreaming state, memory elements may well be reconstituted in an alternative fashion, perhaps randomly,[6] perhaps linked metaphorically,[42] perhaps combined into composite context memories.[49] All of these possibilities may be true to some extent; elements may be activated as a function of emotional concerns[50] but with the possible introduction of some pseudo-random and incompatible associations. The net effect of this organization is to create novel, nonaversive contexts that facilitate fear extinction, particularly under conditions of heightened stress activation. In this way, the authors suggest that dreaming represents an endogenous form of self-correction or equilibration.[51]

An early conceptualization of fear memory organization referred to as fear memory structures[52,53] may help to understand the production of DD. Foa and Kozak[52] describe fear memory structures as networks of information that unite memory elements about (1) a feared stimulus situation (stimulus elements), (2) physiologic, verbal, and behavioral responses to that situation (response elements), and (3) the meaning of these stimuli and responses (meaning elements). During waking, fear memory structures bias the interpretation of new information by enhancing sensitivity and attention to a structure's stimulus elements, thus ensuring the allocation of more cognitive resources to the processing of this new information. Further, activation of these structures interfere with access to resources necessary for competing tasks, as exemplified by the response deficits shown by patients with PTSD on the emotional Stroop task.[54,55]

The construct of fear memory structures has been validated in some respects however, whereas the internal coherence of fear memory structures was believed to be modified or weakened by the introduction of incompatible elements, thus alleviating associated pathologic symptoms.[52] Recent work in experimental psychopathology suggests that these structures may be replaced by the more neurologically specific concept of extinction memories that inhibit fear memories.[56–58]

During dreaming, fear memories seem to vary in how completely and coherently their stimulus and response elements are expressed. Although minimal activation of these structures may trigger a mild anxiety dream in which a limited number of stimulus or response elements are activated, more extensive activation would result in a more intense, nontraumatic nightmare. Under conditions of minimal activation, a few fear memory elements may be expressed in relative isolation and in no coherent order, that is, as common residues. With extensive activation, more elements may be expressed and their order more veridical, rendering the form of the fear memory more easily identifiable from the nightmare's theme. From this model it is predicted that individuals with particularly problematic and coherent fear memories, including persons with specific phobias, ongoing interpersonal difficulties or other current sources of stress, should experience more recurrent dreams and dream themes.

When the level of waking stress reaches extreme levels as in trauma exposure, the fear memory elements may be activated globally and in a highly coherent manner resulting in a nightmare that reproduces the extreme memory with appropriate fear context, bodily reactions and, cognitive interpretations. This type of comprehensive activation is illustrated by PTSD nightmares that seem to replay large portions of the original trauma.[59] Between mild anxiety dreams and intense PTSD nightmares are various types of dysphoric dreams and nightmares that have fear memory elements either alone or in combination and with varying degrees of organization. Examples include dreams or nightmares with recurring objects, characters and themes,[60] typical dream themes,[46] and story- and script-like structures.[61] This ensemble of emotional imagery processes constituting fear memories most likely underlies a variety of clinical conditions characterized by anxiety and fear, such as panic disorder, phobia, and PTSD[57,62] as well as dysphoric dreams and nightmares.

Memory Element Recombination

The second set of processes, responsible for the continuous assembly of memory elements into a constant flow of dream imagery, was termed "condensation"[1,3] and described as the merging of several separate (although motivationally linked) images into a single image. The authors propose that a similar type of reorganization that produces new image contexts during dreaming, much like the remapping of conjunctive representations under control of the hippocampus, occurs during the waking state. During dreaming, conjunctive representations are rendered into virtual simulations or here-and-now illusions[40] to maximize their effect on the amygdala, which favors perceptual, rather than imaginal, stimuli.[63] They are recombined or remapped to introduce elements that are incompatible with existing fear memories, thus facilitating (among other functions) the acquisition or maintenance of extinction memories. The latter inhibit fear memories and consequently, alleviate affect load. Recombinations of memory elements give dreams at once their alien and their familiar quality. Three features of recombination are especially pertinent to the pathology of DDs.

Unlikely combinations

The first is the de novo conjunctions of features, many of which produce dream experience that seems bizarre, incongruous, or incompatible with waking-life experience. Bizarreness is frequent in dreams[64–66] and dreams are significantly more bizarre than waking daydreams.[67] Although

a widely accepted explanation for bizarreness is still lacking, 1 possibility is that bizarreness reflects the relative inactivity of dorsolateral prefrontal executive functioning during REM sleep.[6] Another possibility is that REM sleep selectively permits weakly associated (and thus possibly disjunctive) memory elements to become associated.[68] Regardless, the authors propose that the unlikely combinations of disparate memory elements facilitate acquisition and maintenance of conditioned fear memories and thus of fear responding. Bizarreness may be an inevitable consequence of this mechanism and we would expect to see higher levels of bizarreness in dreams of individuals with high affect load. As this question has not been directly investigated, it remains unknown whether nightmares are more or less bizarre than non-nightmare dreams in this specific sense of recombined elements. To the extent that nightmares replay fear memories or possess recurrent elements they would seem to be less, not more, organizationally bizarre. Further empirical investigation of the organizational coherence of nightmares and normal dreams among individuals suffering from frequent nightmares or from conditions marked by high fear coherence in waking states, such as PTSD or specific phobias, could help elucidate these mechanisms.

Fear memory templates

A second salient feature of recombination is the organizing influence of fear memory and other emotional memory structures. Although they are not usually expressed fully as memory replays, fear memories may act as organizing templates that structure dreams and within which other isolated and frequently incompatible memory elements are ordered and interrelated. As a result, fear-producing stimuli and their physiologic responses will be repeatedly paired with alternative, nonaversive contexts and thus extinguished gradually over time. Although the specific nature of such a mechanism remains speculative, phenomenological features of dream organization belie their presence. On the one hand, fear memories may assume a habitual easily recognized form and express a consistent emotional content in the dream, such as with themes of public nudity, being late, or being pursued.[69] Such themes recur frequently and are associated with diminished psychological well-being until they cease, at which time well-being is high.[12,30] On the other hand, fear memories may portray novel organizations in which a skeletal structure incorporates many unexpected elements, such as an interpersonal attack scenario that introduces many unanticipated characters and produces many unusual consequences. The latter type of dream has been labeled as problem-solving and found to be associated with emotional adaptation.[7,70] Fear extinction is more likely to be associated with the latter type of dream and less likely to be associated with the former, although again, there is no research that addresses this issue directly. One useful line of investigation would be to compare organizational coherence of the dreams, nightmares, and daytime narratives of individuals who have frequent nightmares and report high or low levels of accompanying distress to determine whether memory organization corresponds to waking emotional reactivity. Because fear memories are purportedly responsible for the nonconscious detection of threat, it would also be informative to investigate whether individuals with high nightmare distress perform similar to individuals with anxiety disorders or PTSD on an affective backward masking paradigm or the emotional color-word Stroop test.

Reality simulation

A third important feature of dream imagery recombination is that the new image sequences consist, for the most part, of lifelike simulations of first-person reality. Memory elements are recombined on various levels of organization (eg, perceptual, schematic, thematic, symbolic) to produce coherent, continuous simulations of waking-life experience. Functionally, reconstituting disparate memory elements into virtual simulations may facilitate the creation or strengthening of new memory links and aid in the simulation of threats to species survival, thus optimizing off-line rehearsal of behavioral avoidance responses.[71,72] Thus, reality mimesis ensures that fear memories are processed in a phenomenological medium similar to that in which they were first formed. This process allows for the modification or integration of disturbing emotions during dreaming[8,42] in a fashion analogous to that induced by exposure therapy for waking-state fear-based disorders.[52] The finding that imagery rehearsal is highly effective in reducing recurrent nightmares in individuals with PTSD[73] is consistent with this formulation.

Emotional Expression

There is disagreement on whether emotions drive the selection of dream contents[42,74] or whether they arise later, in reaction to these contents.[75] Our view is that both occur in a progressive interactive expression of fear memories. Because stimulus and response elements are often encoded in a single fear memory,[76] activation of 1 type of element should activate the other. The notion of fear extinction implies a mechanism that produces a mimesis of the waking perception of emotional events, that is, in which stimulus elements preferentially lead to activation of response elements. This ordering maximizes the involvement of the amygdala, which responds preferentially to perceptual stimuli, and thus facilitates regulation of affect load. Emotional expression during dreaming is integral in dreaming's function of fear extinction. The emotions appearing in normal dreams are predominantly dysphoric (eg, two-thirds of normal dreams[60,77] with fear being by far the most prevalent[69]), which is consistent with this suggestion, as is the frequent occurrence of nondistressing bad dreams and nightmares. The authors consider normal dysphoric dreams, bad dreams, and nondistressing, nontraumatic nightmares to be related in this respect. The variable intensity of fear expression in these types of dreams may simply reflect variations in the strength or efficacy of the hypothesized fear extinction function, which is presumed to vary in step with an individual's day-to-day emotional requirements. In contrast, more severe nightmares, such as nontraumatic nightmares with high distress, PTSD nightmares, and extreme PTSD nightmares, are assumed to be shaped additionally by the presence of additional waking distress and/or previous trauma.

NIGHTMARES ARE PATHOLOGIC EXPRESSIONS OF FEAR MEMORIES
Pathogenic Changes Common to All Nightmares

Although fear memories are considered to be a normal phenomenon of human memory, they become pathologic when (1) they are highly coherent and resistant to extinction, and (2) they contain an excessive number of response elements.[52,78] The authors propose that individual vulnerability (ie, high levels of affect load and/or affect distress) interacts with the neurophysiologic state of REM sleep to favor the activation during nightmares of highly coherent fear memories, akin to those occurring in waking, fear-based pathologic conditions. Accordingly, the authors propose that nightmare-related fear memories are highly resistant to extinction, overly weighted with response elements (usually involving escape or avoidance) and, in more severe instances, corrupted by affect distress.

Increased resistance to extinction is reflected in several possible pathologic events. First, during dream formation there may be a marked bias to activate complete fear memories rather than isolated elements of fear memories. Traumatic memories in particular preserve their structural coherence,[53] perhaps as a result of conditions of heightened arousal during encoding, and thereby enter dreams as apparent replays of the original trauma. This replay is accompanied by a sense of perceptual reinstatement and distressing emotions. Novel configurations, including incompatible elements, are thus less likely to be introduced and thus less able to permit acquisition of new extinction memories. Second, the fear memory may simply resist activation altogether. Because availability of a fear memory is a prerequisite for the successful acquisition of an extinction memory,[52,53] a lack of extinction may occur if the fear memory is not fully activated either during dreaming or later, during the waking state. Awakening from a nightmare may cut short fear memory activation and thereby prevent extinction. In addition, the awakening may actually strengthen the fear by serving as an avoidance response. Similarly, avoiding the recall of nightmares on awakening may prevent the eventual extinction of its underlying fear memory.

Increase in fear memory response elements is reflected in several indicators: an increase in the frequency and intensity of motor imagery in nightmares (eg, escaping, defending oneself, fighting, attempting to scream); increased activation of the sleep state as signaled by physiologic measures (eg, heightened autonomic arousal); and the overt expression of sleep behaviors, such as moving in bed, speaking, and emoting. These response elements are often the identifiable correlates of distress that individuals report experiencing during and following their nightmares. A preponderance of response elements may result from a failure of recombinatory processes to limit the number of response elements that are activated and introduced into the narrative.

The production of emotions during dreaming is compounded by the facilitating influence of high levels of waking affect distress. Affect distress elements may become incorporated into an individual's fear memories and other emotional structures such that, when a fear memory is activated, emotional responses will come to include expressions of distress as well as fear. An individual high in affect distress will therefore experience distress whenever certain fear memories are activated either during a nightmare or later in the day, when the nightmare is recalled. The distress experienced may even lead to further, similar nightmare episodes with recurrent themes. This cyclical process is consistent with the finding that intrusive imagery facilitates the release of stress hormones that heightens affect distress and potentiates further intrusive imagery.[79,80] Affect distress may

thereby contribute to the pathologic portrait of an individual's nightmare disorder, including its cyclical nature.

Pathogenic Changes in Nontraumatic Nightmares

Nightmares that are nontraumatic and associated with low waking distress are produced by an intensification of the memory element activation/recombination mechanisms related to normal dreaming and modulated by levels of waking stress (affect load). The authors propose that affect load increases with short-term accumulations of interpersonal conflicts, current affective memory demands, and emotional reactions to transitory stressors. Affect load interacts primarily with the stimulus and contextual elements of fear memories such that high affect load may disrupt activation and recombination of dreamed stimuli, rather than responses. This may have the effect of producing recurrent, typical, bizarre, or macabre imagery with mild anxiety or fear, but not distress. Dreams with little emotional activation may be associated with greater fear memory resistance to extinction than more emotional dreams and nightmares.

Nontraumatic nightmares with high waking distress involve affect distress mechanisms in addition to fear memories and affect load mechanisms. As mentioned earlier, affect distress influences primarily the response elements of fear memories such that subjects high on this trait respond with more subjective upset during and following their nightmares. Thus, the activation of nightmare-related fear memories of individuals high in affect distress may have inadvertent effects during the waking state, such as the stimulation of various conditioned expectancies and biases for the recall and perception of fear-relevant stimuli. Although these processes have not been investigated directly in frequent nightmare individuals, there is abundant evidence that (1) negatively arousing memories are recalled with greater clarity than neutral ones, particularly for memories of high personal significance[81]; and (2) individuals with vivid imagistic abilities, a quality that characterizes frequent nightmare individuals, demonstrate heightened autonomic and emotional activation when presented with fear-relevant stimuli.[82]

Pathogenic Changes in Traumatic Nightmares

Trauma is hypothesized to cause an underlying fear memory to become firmly entrenched and highly resistant to extinction. This may mean that there is a diminution of recombinatory dream elements and thereby an increase of fear memory coherence. Degree of fear memory coherence is believed to underlie the severity of PTSD symptoms.[62] The authors suggest that fear memory resistance to extinction is responsible for the finding that PTSD nightmare content seems to replicate the original trauma.[59] A similar process may underlie memory more generally. For example, highly specific autobiographical memories are often associated with higher levels of emotional distress.[53] Thus, in contrast to the variable progression of dysphoric imagery seen in nontraumatic nightmares, PTSD nightmares are more likely to be realistic and predictable as a result of the activation of structurally coherent fear memories.

Second, in the case of traumatic nightmares, the response elements of underlying fear memories may be especially salient and amplified by affect distress. This is suggested by the presence of several sleep-related hyperarousal symptoms, including increased awakenings, wake after sleep onset and insomnia, as well as nightmares in stages other than REM sleep and at times other than the habitual last third of the night; for example, stage 2 nightmares occurring early in the sleep episode.[83] It is also suggested by the expression of motor activity in sleep, including more frequent REM-related twitches in leg muscles, more periodic leg movements in sleep in all stages, more frequent gross body movements, and more REM-related motor activity and vocalizations.[84] That PTSD is comorbid with many cases of REM sleep behavior disorder,[85] which is characterized by motorically active dreams and diminished REM sleep muscle atonia, further implicates excessive response elements and distress in PTSD nightmare formation.

The spectrum of dysphoric dreams that includes nontraumatic and traumatic nightmares may be attributed to interactions between fear memories, short-term accumulations of affect load, and a pathogenic distress diathesis in vulnerable individuals. Fear memory coherence and resistance to extinction may be a factor common to all types of dysphoric dreaming, whereas affect distress distinguishes pathologic from nonpathologic nightmares. In addition to the pathologic sleep changes described earlier, it is also highly likely that these processes interact in various ways during waking states, and that sleep- and waking-state interactions among processes also occur. To illustrate, phobic individuals who selectively process phobic threat cues and focus narrowly on stimuli that activate their underlying phobia-relevant fear memories may apply the same acquired encoding biases to selectively scan their dream imagery for threats and to reflect

on their recalled nightmares with a similar narrow focus. As a result, such individuals may experience nightmares as more threatening and distressing than do other types of individuals and may be more likely to misattribute their endogenous imagery to actual environmental threats; a type of source-monitoring deficit documented for normal dreaming.[86] Further, the physiologic conditions of REM sleep may facilitate this process. Thus, nightmares can be likened to false alarm responses, in a manner similar to the false alarm responses of panic disorder.[87]

NEURAL LEVEL EXPLANATION: A BRAIN NETWORK FOR FEAR IMAGERY

Recent research on the brain correlates of emotion, fear memory, PTSD, and human sleep and dreaming, has begun to clarify the nature of normal and posttraumatic emotional processing during sleep. Much of this work suggests that DDs may result from disturbances in a network of brain regions controlling the processing of fear and distress, namely a brain network of limbic, paralimbic, and prefrontal regions that constitutes the control center for several emotional processes, including the perception and representation of emotional stimuli and the expression and regulation of emotional responses. Although still preliminary, these structures likely include the amygdala and its medial prefrontal cortex extension, as well as the hippocampal complex and its anterior cingulate cortex extension.[88,89]

The authors suggest that the 4 designated brain regions operate synergistically as part of a larger emotional control structure, which in turn influences other perceptual, cognitive, memorial, and affective brain events. These conclusions are based on several anatomic and functional considerations. First, these regions are interconnected anatomically and functionally.[90] Amygdala, in particular, is massively connected to the other regions in a reciprocal fashion[91] and all 4 regions are functionally connected to sensory, motor, and autonomic brain regions, and are thus well-suited to mediate higher cognitive functions, behaviors, and affective responses. For example, the hippocampus and amygdala are now considered to be integral in basic dream production.[6,40] In addition, all 4 neural regions are crucial in the formation and regulation of normal emotions, fear in particular,[63] with the amygdala being central in this process, likely by virtue of its connections with hypothalamic structures.[91] The medial prefrontal cortex and hippocampus are critical for the acquisition and memory of conditioned fear and fear extinction, whereas the anterior cingulated cortex (ACC) seems to be crucial for mediating affect distress.[92] These regions are associated with state and trait individual differences in emotional responding, thus allowing for future direct tests of cross-state continuity between waking functioning and neural and structural changes in the brain. Not surprisingly, these regions are also implicated in emotion-based disorders including, but not limited to, anxiety disorders (generalized anxiety, social anxiety, phobia, panic, obsessive-compulsive disorder), mood disorders (depression, bipolar disorder), personality disorders (borderline, psychopathy) and most importantly for our discussion, PTSD. Although the exact neurophysiologic mechanisms underlying emotion-based personality attributes and anxiety disorders remain a topic of intensive investigation, recent work in PTSD brain functioning is instructive for application to the pathogenesis of DD. One leading hypothesis for PTSD formation[89,93] is that symptoms result from a hyper-responsivity of the amygdala to threat stimuli, leading to exaggerated symptoms of arousal and distress, coupled with a failure of the other brain regions (hippocampus, medial prefrontal cortex, ACC) to adequately dampen this activation. A similar pathologic mechanism may explain the generation of DDs with the amygdala becoming increasingly responsive to fear-related memory elements portrayed in the dream, while its regulation by medial prefrontal cortex, hippocampus, and ACC is disturbed in some way. Severe and traumatic nightmares are particularly affected by disturbance of the ACC, which amplifies the intensity of the distress within the actual dream and on awakening from the dream. Imaging studies have also shown that activity levels in the 4 AMPHAC regions increase during REM sleep higher than levels seen in either wakefulness or non-REM sleep.[4,6,94,95]

SUMMARY

The AMPHAC/AND network is a vital component of the physiologic infrastructure of normal dreaming and likely influences the shaping of emotional imagery during normal and DD. By its endemic nature, dreaming is a naturally occurring self-regulatory process that may operate much like the emotional processing and habituation or desensitization that occurs during exposure therapy.[51,96] Thus, the nature and quality of REM sleep in particular likely interacts with these brain regions in the formation of dream imagery to facilitate the reduction or even elimination of fear-based memories in an ongoing attempt at achieving emotional homeostasis and optimize survival function.

REFERENCES

1. Freud S. The interpretation of dreams. New York: Basic Books; 1955.
2. Gilboa A, Shalev AY, Laor L, et al. Functional connectivity of the prefrontal cortex and the amygdala in posttraumatic stress disorder. Biol Psychiatry 2004;55:263–72.
3. Jung CG. Dreams: the collected works of C.G. Jung. Princeton (NJ): Princeton University Press; 1974.
4. Maquet P, Péters J-M, Aerts J, et al. Functional neuroanatomy of human rapid-eye-movement sleep and dreaming. J Cogn Neurosci 1996;383:163–6.
5. McGaugh JL. The amygdala modulates the consolidation of memories of emotionally arousing experiences. Annu Rev Neurosci 2004;27:1–28.
6. Hobson JA, Pace-Schott E, Stickgold R. Dreaming and the brain: towards a cognitive neuroscience of conscious states. Behav Brain Sci 2000;23:793–842.
7. Kramer M. The selective mood regulatory function of dreaming: an update and revision. In: Moffitt A, Kramer M, Hoffmann R, editors. The functions of dreaming. Albany (NY): State University of New York; 1993. p. 139–96.
8. Cartwright R. Dreaming as a mood regulation system. In: Kryger MH, Roth T, Dement WC, editors. Principles and practice of sleep medicine. 4th edition. Philadelphia: Elsevier Saunders; 2005. p. 565–72.
9. Cartwright RD. Affect and dream work from an information processing point of view. J Mind Behav 1986;7:411–27.
10. Vogel GW. A review of REM sleep deprivation. Arch Gen Psychiatry 1975;32:749–61.
11. Cartwright RD, Kravitz HM, Eastman CI, et al. REM latency and the recovery from depression: getting over divorce. Am J Psychiatry 1991;148:1530–5.
12. Brown RJ, Donderi DC. Dream content and self-reported well-being among recurrent dreamers, past-recurrent dreamers, and nonrecurrent dreamers. J Pers Soc Psychol 1986;50:612–23.
13. Cartwright RD. The nature and function of repetitive dreams: a survey and speculation. Psychiatry 1979;42:131–7.
14. Zadra A, Desjardins S, Marcotte E. Evolutionary function of dreams: a test of the threat simulation theory in recurrent dreams. Conscious Cogn 2006;15:450–63.
15. Bremner JD, Vythilingam M, Vermetten E, et al. Neural correlates of declarative memory for emotionally valenced words in women with posttraumatic

stress disorder related to early childhood sexual abuse. Biol Psychiatry 2003;53:879–89.

16. Breslau N, Chilcoat HD, Kessler RC, et al. Previous exposure to trauma and PTSD effects of subsequent trauma: results from the Detroit area survey of trauma. Am J Psychiatry 1999;156:902–7.

17. Breslau N, Roth T, Rosenthal L, et al. Sleep disturbance and psychiatric disorders: a longitudinal epidemiological study of young adults. Biol Psychiatry 1996;39:411–8.

18. Ford DE, Kamerow DB. Epidemiologic study of sleep disturbances and psychiatric disorders: an opportunity for prevention? JAMA 1989;262:1479–84.

19. Walker MP, Stickhold R. Sleep, memory and plasticity. Annu Rev Psychol 2006;57:139–66.

20. Levin R, Nielsen T. Disturbed dreaming, posttraumatic stress disorder, and affect distress: a review and neurocognitive model. Psychol Bull 2007;133:482–528.

21. Levin R, Nielsen T. Nightmares, bad dreams, and emotion dysregulation. Curr Dir Psychol Sci 2009;18:84–8.

22. Liberzon I, Phan KL. Brain-imaging studies of posttraumatic stress disorder. CNS Spectr 2003;8:641–50.

23. Nielsen T, Levin R. Nightmares: a new neurocognitive model. Sleep Med Rev 2007;11:295–310.

24. Levin R. Sleep and dreaming characteristics of frequent nightmare subjects in a university population. Dreaming 1994;4:127–37.

25. Berquier A, Ashton R. Characteristics of the frequent nightmare sufferer. J Abnorm Psychol 1992;101:246–50.

26. Blagrove M, Farmer L, Williams E. The relationship of nightmare frequency and nightmare distress to well-being. J Sleep Res 2004;13:129–36.

27. Hartmann E, Russ D, Oldfield M, et al. Who has nightmares? The personality of the lifelong nightmare sufferer. Arch Gen Psychiatry 1987;44:49–56.

28. Levin R, Fireman G. Nightmare prevalence, nightmare distress, and self-reported psychological disturbance. Sleep 2002;25:205–12.

29. Nielsen T, Levin R. The dimensional nature of disturbed dreaming: reply to Weiss (2007). Psychol Bull 2007;133:533–4.

30. Zadra A, Donderi D. Nightmares and bad dreams: their prevalence and relationship to well-being. J Abnorm Psychol 2000;109:273–81.

31. Nielsen TA, Laberge L, Tremblay R, et al. Development of disturbing dreams during adolescence and their relationship to anxiety symptoms. Sleep 2000;23:727–36.

32. Beauchemin K, Hays P. Prevailing mood, mood changes and dreams in bipolar disorder. J Affect Disord 1995;35:41–9.

33. Belicki K. Nightmare frequency versus nightmare distress: relations to psychopathology and cognitive style. J Abnorm Psychol 1992;101:592–7.

34. Levin R. Ego boundary impairment and thought disorder in frequent nightmare sufferers. Psychoanal Psychol 1990;7:529–43.

35. Mellman TA, David D, Kulick-Bell R, et al. Sleep disturbance and its relationship to psychiatric morbidity after hurricane Andrew. Am J Psychiatry 1995;152:1659–63.

36. Woodward SH, Arsenault NJ, Murray C, et al. Laboratory sleep correlates of nightmare complaint in PTSD inpatients. Biol Psychiatry 2000;48:1081–7.

37. Wood JM, Bootzin RR, Rosenhan D, et al. Effects of the 1989 San Francisco earthquake on frequency and content of nightmares. J Abnorm Psychol 1992;101:219–24.

38. Levin R, Fireman G, Pope A. Disturbed Dreaming. Front Neurosci 2009;3:448–9.

39. Fosse MJ, Fosse R, Hobson JA, et al. Dreaming and episodic memory: a functional dissociation? J Cogn Neurosci 2003;15:1–9.

40. Nielsen TA, Stenstrom P. What are the memory sources of dreaming? Nature 2005;437:34–8.

41. Nielsen TA, Zadra AL. Nightmares and other common dream disturbances. In: Kryger M, Roth N, Dement WC, editors. Principles and practice of sleep medicine. 4th edition. Philadelphia: Elsevier Saunders; 2005. p. 926–35.

42. Hartmann E. Dreams and nightmares: the new theory on the origin and meaning of dreams. New York: Plenum; 1998.

43. Cipolli C, Bolzani R, Tuozzi G, et al. Active processing of declarative knowledge during REM-sleep dreaming. J Sleep Res 2001;10:277–84.

44. Hoelscher TJ, Klinger E, Barta SG. Incorporation of concern and nonconcern-related verbal stimuli into dream content. J Abnorm Psychol 1981;90:88–91.

45. Saredi R, Baylor GW, Meier B, et al. Current concerns and REM-dreams: a laboratory study of dream incubation. Dreaming 1997;7:195–208.

46. Nielsen TA, Kuiken D, Alain G, et al. Immediate and delayed incorporations of events into dreams: further replication and implications for dream function. J Sleep Res 2004;13:327–36.

47. Schacter DL, Tulving E. Memory systems 1994. Cambridge (MA): MIT Press; 1994.

48. Nadel L, Moscovitch M. Hippocampal contributions to cortical plasticity. Neuropharmacology 1998;37:431–9.

49. Johnson JD. REM sleep and the development of context memory. Med Hypotheses 2005;64:499–504.

50. Klinger E. Daydreaming. Using waking fantasy and imagery for self-knowledge and creativity. Los Angeles (CA): Jeremy P. Tarcher; 1990.

51. Walker MP, van der Helm E. Overnight therapy? The role of sleep in emotional brain processing. Psychol Bull 2009;135:731–48.

52. Foa EB, Kozak MJ. Emotional processing of fear: exposure to corrective information. Psychol Bull 1986;99:20–35.

53. Lang PJ. Presidential address, 1978. A bio-informational theory of emotional imagery. Psychophysiology 1979;16:495–512.

54. Foa EB, Feske U, Murdock TB, et al. Processing of threat-related information in rape victims. J Abnorm Psychol 1991;100:156–62.

55. McNally RJ. Experimental approaches to cognitive abnormality in posttraumatic stress disorder. Clin Psychol Rev 1998;18:971–82.

56. Lang PJ, Davis M, Ohman A. Fear and anxiety: animal models and human cognitive psychophysiology. J Affect Disord 2000;61:137–59.

57. Mineka S, Zimbarg R. A contemporary learning theory perspective on the etiology of anxiety disorders: it's not what you thought it was. Am Psychol 2006;61:10–26.

58. Ohman A, Mineka S. Fears, phobias and preparedness: towards an evolved module of fear and fear learning. Psychol Rev 2001;108:483–522.

59. Mellman TA, Pigeon WR. Dreams and nightmares in posttraumatic stress disorder. In: Kryger MH, Roth T, Dement WC, editors. Principles and practice of sleep medicine. 4th edition. Philadelphia: Elsevier Saunders; 2005. p. 573–8.

60. Domhoff GW. Finding meaning in dreams. A quantitative approach. New York: Plenum; 1996.

61. Cipolli C, Bolzani R, Tuozzi G. Story-like organization of dream experience in different periods of REM sleep. J Sleep Res 1998;7:13–9.

62. Foa EB, Meadows EA. Psychosocial treatments for post-traumatic stress disorder: a critical review. Annu Rev Psychol 1997;48:449–80.

63. Phan KL, Wager T, Taylor SF, et al. Functional neuroanatomy of emotion: a meta-analysis of emotion activation studies in PET and fMRI. Neuroimage 2002;16:331–48.

64. Levin R, Livingston G. Concordance between two measures of dream bizarreness. Percept Mot Skills 1991;72:837–8.

65. Revonsuo A, Salmivalli C. A content analysis of bizarre elements in dreams. Dreaming 1995;5:169–87.

66. Rudy JW, Matus-Amat P. The ventral hippocampus supports a memory representation of context and contextual fear conditioning: implications for a unitary function of the hippocampus. Behav Neurosci 2005;119:154–63.

67. Kunzendorf RG, Hartmann E, Cohen R, et al. Bizarreness of the dreams and daydreams reported by individuals with thin and thick boundaries. Dreaming 1997;7:265–71.

68. Stickgold R, Scott L, Rittenhouse C, et al. Sleep-induced changes in associative memory. J Cogn Neurosci 1999;11:182–93.

69. Nielsen TA, Zadra AL, Simard V, et al. The typical dreams of Canadian university students. Dreaming 2003;13:211–35.

70. Cartwright RD. Dreams that work: the relation of dream incorporation to adaptation to stressful events. Dreaming 1991;1:3–9.

71. Stickgold R, Hobson JA, Fosse R, et al. Sleep, learning, and dreams: off-line memory reprocessing. Science 2001;294:1052–7.

72. Revonsuo A. The reinterpretation of dreams: an evolutionary hypothesis of the function of dreaming. Behav Brain Sci 2000;23:877–901.

73. Krakow B, Zadra A. Clinical management of chronic nightmares: imagery rehearsal therapy. Behav Sleep Med 2006;4:45–70.

74. Newell PT, Cartwright RD. Affect and cognition in dreams: a critique of the cognitive role in adaptive dream functioning and support for associative models. Psychiatry 2000;63:34–44.

75. Foulkes D. Dreaming: a cognitive-psychological analysis. Hillsdale (NJ): Lawrence Erlbaum Associates; 1985.

76. Rudy JW, Huff NC, Matus-Amat P. Understanding contextual fear conditioning: insights from a two-process model. Neurosci Biobehav Rev 2004;28:675–85.

77. Hartmann E. We do not dream of the 3 R's: implications for the nature of dreaming mentation. Dreaming 2000;10:103–10.

78. Vrana SR, Cuthbert BN, Lang PJ. Fear imagery and text processing. Psychophysiology 1986;23:247–53.

79. Pitman RK, Orr SP. Psychophysiology of emotional memory networks in posttraumatic stress disorder. In: McGaugh JL, Weinberger NM, Lynch G, editors. Brain and memory: modulation and mediation of neuroplasticity. New York: Oxford University Press; 1995. p. 75–83.

80. Rauch SL, Shin LM, Segal E, et al. Selectively reduced regional cortical volumes in posttraumatic stress disorder. Neuroreport 2003;14:913–6.

81. Ochsner KN. Are affective events richly recollected or simply familiar? The experience and process of recognizing feelings past. J Exp Psychol Gen 2000;129:242–61.

82. Lang PJ, Greenwald MK, Bradley MM, et al. Looking at pictures: affective, facial, visceral, and behavioral reactions. Psychophysiology 1993;30:261–73.

83. van der Kolk B, Blitz R, Burr W, et al. Nightmares and trauma: a comparison of nightmares after combat with lifelong nightmares in veterans. Am J Psychiatry 1984;141:187–90.

84. Lavie P. Sleep disturbances in the wake of traumatic events. N Engl J Med 2001;345:1825–32.

85. Husain AM, Miller PP, Carwile ST. REM sleep behavior disorder: potential relationship to post-traumatic stress disorder. J Clin Neurophysiol 2001;18:148–57.

86. Johnson MK, Kahan TL, Raye CL. Dreams and reality monitoring. J Exp Psychol Gen 1984;113: 329–44.

87. Clark DM. A cognitive model of panic attacks. In: Rachman S, Maser JD, editors. Panic: psychological perspectives. Hillsdale (NJ): Erlbaum; 1988. p. 71–89.

88. Hull AM. Neuroimaging findings in post-traumatic stress disorder. Systematic review. Br J Psychiatry 2002;181:102–10.

89. Nutt DJ, Malizia AL. Structural and functional brain changes in posttraumatic stress disorder. J Clin Psychiatry 2004;65(Suppl 1):11–7.

90. Morgane PJ, Galler JR, Mokler DJ. A review of systems and networks of the limbic forebrain/limbic midbrain. Prog Neurobiol 2005;75:143–60.

91. LeDoux JE. Emotion circuits in the brain. Annu Rev Neurosci 2000;23:155–84.

92. Eisenberger NI, Lieberman MD. Why rejection hurts: a common neural alarm system for physical and social pain. Trends Cogn Sci 2004;8:294–300.

93. Rauchs G, Bertran F, Guillery-Girard B, et al. Consolidation of strictly episodic memories mainly requires rapid eye movement sleep. Sleep 2004; 27:395–401.

94. Braun AR, Balkin TJ, Wesensten NJ, et al. Dissociated pattern of activity in visual cortices and their projections during human rapid eye movement sleep. Science 1998;279:91–5.

95. Nofzinger EA. What can neuroimaging findings tell us about sleep disorders? Sleep Med 2004;5(Suppl 1):S16–22.

96. Hartmann E. Making connections in a safe place: is dreaming psychotherapy? Dreaming 1995;5: 213–28.

The Dream Always Makes New Connections: The Dream is a Creation, Not a Replay

Ernest Hartmann, MD[a,b,*]

KEYWORDS

- Dreams • Dreaming • Connection in dreams
- Dreams as creation • Dream replay • Dream function

Every dream makes new connections, and every dream is a creative product not a replay. This article summarizes evidence that even dreams usually thought of as replays—recurrent or repetitive dreams and post-traumatic stress disorder (PTSD) dreams—turn out to be new creations, rather than replays. It will discuss the implications of this view for the functions of dreaming. The data suggest that dreaming is not involved in the consolidation of memory, but rather in integrating new memories into memory schemes, guided by emotion. This view of dreaming also has implications for making use of dreams in therapy and in self-knowledge.

There is a view that dreaming or at least dreaming in rapid eye movement (REM) sleep involves a replay of material experienced in waking and that therefore dreaming is involved in the consolidation of memory. This view is based in part on the frequent appearance of bits of waking experiences in dreams (day residue) and in part on recent studies showing that in rats, hippocampal place cells fire during REM sleep in a pattern similar to their firing while the rats navigated a maze some hours earlier.[1,2] This article will show that studies of human dream content do not support the idea of replay.

A dream certainly may incorporate events that occur the day or days before the dream (the day

residue). In fact incorporation of daytime material into dreams has been studied in some detail.[3,4] It appears that bits of daytime material found in dreams come especially from the day of the dream, with some evidence suggesting that material from about 1 week before the dream also is favored. I have reported that material from about 2 hours before sleep onset on the day of the dream is the most likely to show up in dreams.[5]

In all of the dream series I have studied, however, the dream does not repeat the waking material, but changes it, combines it, and weaves it into an ongoing story. For instance, consider dream setting; the dream often takes place in a specific spot or town known from waking life, sometimes a place the dreamer has visited or spent time in recently. But just as often the setting is a combination of several places. For example, I often dream of a city that is Boston, but it is also New York. Both are cities that I have lived in and know well. Even if the setting is definitely one city, the more details I remember, the more it seems that it is not exactly the same as the city I know in waking life. And what happens in the setting is invariably different from what happened in waking life.

The characters in the dream may be people one knows, or people one has seen recently, or strangers, or people who seem familiar but the

[a] Department of Psychiatry, Tufts University School of Medicine, Boston, MA, USA
[b] 27 Clark Street, Newton, MA 02459, USA
* 27 Clark Street, Newton, MA 02459.
E-mail address: ehdream@aol.com

sleeper is not sure who they are. And the characters are notoriously shifty, they are sometimes two people at once, or one person, but he is not quite right; there is something different about him. He looks a bit like someone else.

In terms of actions or occurrences in the dream, a dream does sometimes refer to or pick up something that happened recently, most often on the day of the dream. There is never (or rather almost never to be on the safe side) a replay of a waking event, even if it is a powerful or emotional event, even a trauma.

My collaborators and I have studied many series of dreams after trauma.[6] The author and colleagues saw no dreams that replayed the traumatic events or other events exactly as they occurred. They recently completed a systematic study of dreams before and after September 11, 2001. Forty-four people who had been keeping dream journals for years each sent 20 dreams from their records—the last 10 recorded before September 11, 2001, and the first 10 after.[7] The 880 dreams were examined and scored on a blind basis. The most important finding of the study was that the intensity of the central image (based on a reliable rating scale[6]) was significantly higher in the after dreams. There was no difference in dream length, dream-likeness, vividness, and several other measures. Most important for the present argument is that not a single one of the 880 dreams (440 of them after September 11, 2001) involved planes hitting tall buildings or similar scenarios, even though all the participants had seen these events many times on television (and it was clearly an emotionally important experience). No scenes were pictured that were even close to the actual attacks. So even something as striking as the September 11, 2001, attacks generally does not appear in dreams as a replay.

But are there not exceptions? For instance, are there not many reports of recurrent dreams, repetitive dreams, and especially repetitive dreams of trauma (PTSD dreams)? Do these dreams not replay frightening events from the dreamer's life? Recurrent dreams indeed have been the subject of numerous studies.[8–10] Usually recurrent dreams are frightening dreams most often beginning in childhood. These dreams usually are really dreams about a recurrent theme. The dreams mentioned in the studies cited previously and dreams I have surveyed are never or almost never precisely repetitive dreams. And they do not replay waking life events, although they may incorporate bits of material, for instance from a traumatic childhood. The general theme of the dreams is the same each time, but there are usually changes in the dream as the dreamer's life and emotional state change.

A patient in psychoanalysis provided an especially clear series of nightmares, which appeared to reflect her mental state. This very intelligent young woman reported having recurrent dreams. She described a series of dreams going back many years, which involved sharks or shark-like monsters chasing her in the ocean. In one dream she was held captive by shark–monsters that were going to torture or kill her. The details varied, but the dangerous shark theme was constant. These dreams seemed to occur especially when some important change was happening in her life. They also occurred several times during her psychoanalysis, at the times when she was unsure of herself and when she seemed to be re-experiencing childhood fears and childhood helplessness. Over the course of several years she made gradual progress in understanding her life and overcoming her fears. During this time she had several more dreams of sharks, but the sharks gradually became less terrifying than before. She no longer woke up scared whenever she dreamt of a shark. Finally, at a time when she was finishing her treatment, when her life and work were going well, she had one final dream of a shark. This time she was at a swimming pool rather than in the ocean. A friendly little shark came out of the swimming pool right next to her. She patted it on the head and it curled up at her feet like a pet dog.[11] Obviously the recurrent dreams here kept the theme of a shark but changed to reflect her emotional state. They were not exactly repetitive, and obviously, they were not replays of actual events.

Thus, recurrent dreams are usually not exactly repetitive dreams. Does this mean that there is no such thing as a repetitive dream? No, there are repetitive dreams, although they are not frequent. There is in fact one situation in which the same dream is experienced again and again, the post-traumatic dreams that occur in PTSD. These post-traumatic nightmares are indeed one diagnostic feature in making the diagnosis of PTSD according to the *Diagnostic and Statistical Manual of Mental Disorders (Fourth Edition, DSM-IV)*.[12] I have studied such dreams both in my research work and in clinical work with veterans and others. Even these truly repetitive dreams, sometimes described as replays of waking events, turn out on examination to be creations, not simple replays of waking events.

Often the veteran suffering from PTSD says, "The dream is just the way it was... I was in a foxhole...noise all around me... a shell explodes... just the way it was!" But in all the cases I have examined in detail, the dream is not just the way it was. There is at least one important change.

For instance, one of the most common dreams in Vietnam veterans goes something like this, "I'm back there in the foxhole. Just the way it was. There's noise all around. A shell explodes right in front of me. I scream, and I'm dying as I wake up." What actually happened was that a shell exploded and killed the man's buddy, his best friend, who was in the foxhole with him, or somewhere nearby. The dream does not simply replay the event. It adds a slight but important change: the dreamer himself is dying rather than his buddy. This appears to be a replay of the events, but slightly altered, probably by an emotion, the emotion known as survivor guilt. The dreamer feels guilty that he survived while his buddy died. Thus, even these so-called repetitive post-traumatic dreams involve the making of new connections. And the connections are guided by emotion, which is consider a basic characteristic of dreaming in general.[13–15] These dreams too turn out to be creations, not simple replays of events.

The most dramatic example in my experience occurred in a Vietnam veteran who suffered for years from PTSD. He had been a medical corpsman, and his job consisted of working just behind the front lines, loading wounded soldiers and body bags off of a helicopter returning from the lines. His job involved getting the wounded men to the right places for treatment and properly identifying dead soldiers in the body bags. The most traumatic event he experienced occurred just after a serious battle. He was opening body bags one after another and found his best buddy in the last body bag he opened. He has dreamt about his experience over and over again for many years. He indeed does have a repetitive dream, which occurs unaltered time after time. In reporting the dream he says, "I open up the body bags one by one, I zip open the last body bag. The body inside is me, and I wake up screaming." Obviously he has taken a serious traumatic incident and changed it slightly in his dreams so that it is he rather his friend who has died. One can see this dream as picturing terror and vulnerability, but also guilt, related to his having survived while his buddy died. So even here, in a repetitive PTSD dream, something new has been added. The repetitive dream is not simply a replay of waking events. My colleagues and I have studied many traumatic dreams with a very similar structure.

DREAMING IS HYPERCONNECTIVE

Returning to dreams in general, my conclusion is that new connections always are involved. Indeed dreams are hyperconnective. Actually, there is little disagreement on this point. Dreams obviously throw together a great deal of material in one's mind. Everyone remembers dreaming about a person who is like A but also somewhat like B. I often have dreams set in a house that is partly my current house and partly a previous house. Also, as mentioned previously, I am often in a city that is both Boston and New York.

Freud called the first and most prominent mechanism of the dreamwork "condensation," and he had exactly this hyperconnectivity in mind. When analyzing a dream by free association, one pulls apart the elements of the condensation, looks for associations to each part, and gradually tries to reconstruct the latent dream thoughts, the thoughts underlying the dream. Freud's view was that most or all parts of a dream are overdetermined; they are produced by the coming together of several underlying thoughts.

Biologically oriented researchers also often speak of hyperconnectivity. What they have in mind, however, is throwing things together randomly. They usually consider dreaming to be a state of random activation, exciting many parts of the forebrain, and thus throwing together all sorts of material from the memory stores.[16]

Thus, basically there is wide agreement that dreams are hyperconnective, and that the connections are broader and looser than in waking. I believe that this broader and looser connectivity is an extremely important aspect of the nature of dreaming. Dreaming brings together things that are kept apart in waking.

First, on an anecdotal or clinical level, here is an example that clarifies this connectivity. I have heard the following dream from six different women, including both friends and patients. The dream goes something like this: "A powerful vivid dream. I dreamt about my boyfriend 'Jim,' but then he turned into someone else; he seemed to be my father."

Each of the six women continued:

"on waking up I thought about it and I realized Jim really is a lot like my father. He's… (and they would enumerate a number of similarities between their boyfriend and their father). But you know something fascinating. I had never thought of it before! I had never noticed the obvious similarities until I had this dream!"

I think this provides a significant insight into the way the human mind works. Apparently these women kept their thoughts, feelings, and memories about Jim in one part of their minds—one compartment—and their thoughts, feelings about their father in another. The compartments were entirely separate while they were awake. It took a dream to make the connection, to cross the boundary from one compartment to another. In other words while awake, one's thinking stays in a groove, or a rut. One keeps thinking along the same straight lines. In dreaming, one can jump out of the groove. This is responsible for people sometimes having all sorts of new insights based on their dreams, and occasionally making new discoveries or creating new works of art.

There have been a few attempts to demonstrate this broader and looser connectivity experimentally. Some years ago I showed, in a small unpublished study, that people given a standard word association test shortly after being awakened from REM sleep produced more distant associations than when awakened from non-REM (NREM) sleep. The idea was that the broader, looser functioning of the mind and brain in REM-sleep dreaming would continue for a few minutes after awakening. Fiss and colleagues, along the same lines, reported that waking fantasy was more "unlikely" and "imagistic" after awakenings from REM as compared with NREM-sleep.[17]

Stickgold and colleagues performed a much more elegant version of this study and obtained significant results. They measured the time in milliseconds required for subjects to recognize close or strong associations between pairs of words, versus distant or weak associations. They found that after REM sleep awakenings the weak associations were made more quickly.[18]

With a slightly different approach, the author and colleagues performed a large questionnaire study investigating the view that dreaming makes connections more broadly and loosely than waking and avoids tightly structured, overlearned material.[19] They did this by investigating the extent to which one reads, writes, and calculates in dreams. The author and colleagues considered reading, writing, and arithmetic to represent the most tightly structured overlearned portions of human mental functioning.

First, two scorers examined a series of 456 dreams for any mention of reading a text, writing, typing, or calculating. The scorers agreed perfectly and found no reading, no writing, and one possible instance of calculating. Second, the author and colleagues obtained 240 completed questionnaires that asked several good dream recallers about any reading, writing, and arithmetic in their dreams. They also were asked to rate the relative prominence of six activities (walking, writing, talking with friends, reading, sexual activity, typing) in their waking and dreaming lives. The results were clear-cut. On the broad questions, the respondents reported almost no reading, writing, and calculating. On the relative prominence scales reading, writing, and typing were scored far more prominent in waking than in dreaming, whereas, walking, talking with friends, and sexual activity were scored almost as frequent in dreaming as in waking.

THE DREAM AS A CREATIVE PRODUCT: IS A DREAM SIMILAR TO A WORK OF ART?

As has been seen, a dream always makes new connections. Thus a dream can be considered to be a creative product, and in this sense, a dream is somewhat similar to a work of art. Creating a work of art has been defined in many ways, usually emphasizing that old materials are put together in a new way, and put together in a new way influenced by the artist's emotion.[20] This is not a random process of course; materials are put together in a way that expresses an underlying emotion or emotional theme. In other words, art in general can be thought of as making new connections guided by emotions, which is exactly the way dreaming has been described.[13,14]

Film and painting are sometimes consciously based on dreams, and films often are considered the most oneiric (dreamlike) of the arts. But other arts are based on dreams also. Several writers have attributed their poems or stories to dreams. Robert Louis Stevenson famously stated that his stories came to him directly from his dreams invented by his "committee of sleep."[21] Some have understood this to mean that the stories actually came to him word for word in his dreams. From my experience, and the study on reading and writing mentioned above, I consider this very unlikely. I would suggest that a powerful image came to him in a dream, for instance, a well-dressed physician turning into a monster (not an uncommon sort of nightmare image), and he then proceeded to fill in the details and write *Dr Jekyll and Mr Hyde* using his well-developed novelistic skills.

I believe that poems too often have a powerful central image. In fact what T.S. Eliot has called the "objective correlative" of a poem is strikingly similar to what has been called the central image of a dream. For instance, consider the image that Eliot himself cites, when discussing the objective correlative, from his poem "The Love Song of J. Alfred Prufrock:"[22]

I should have been a pair of ragged claws
Scuttling across the floors of silent seas.

This powerful image, occurring starkly in the middle of the poem, pictures the social shyness of the narrator who feels uncomfortable with the women who "come and go speaking of a Michelangelo." Here the image obviously pictures an emotional state or emotional concern as occurs in dreaming.[13,14]

In this sense the dream is actually similar to a poem or other work of art, although of course the dream seldom produces a complete work but rather the beginnings of a work of art. As is well known, the new connections in dreams also can help to produce new works of art (and of science). Numerous examples are cited in Barrett, *The Committee of Sleep*.[23] Of course this only happens when the mind is prepared, and I would add that the problem must be an emotional concern of the dreamer. Elias Howe, who had a dream that led to the design of the sewing machine, had been trying for a long time to invent a workable model, so the problem was immensely important to him.

Some may consider this discussion of a dream related to a work of art as somewhat far-fetched. But one arrives at a similar conclusion about the dream as a creative product if one starts by examining the development of dreaming in childhood. Foulkes has done the only careful laboratory-based study on the development of dreaming in childhood.[24,25] His somewhat surprising conclusion is that mature dreaming involving the dreamer's self, other characters, and interactions between people develops only slowly between the ages of 5 and 10 years. In summarizing his work, he noted that dreaming develops in children along with the development of active imagination and storytelling. He concludes:

"dreaming is not at all a form of perception, or 'passive seeing.' It is active imagining," which is a separate function that develops slowly over the years of childhood.[24] "Dreaming is a creative recombination of memories and knowledge, Dreaming is not simple replay of global units from our past experience."

Thus, starting with the development of dreaming in childhood leads to the same conclusion: that dreaming is a creative product.

IMPLICATIONS FOR THE FUNCTIONS OF DREAMING

As of now, the functions of dreaming are unknown. This is not surprising since we do not even know the functions of sleep with certainty. I believe, however, the creative connection making of

dreams that has been discussed previously does lead to a possible functional role. I suggest that dreaming has a function and that it involves weaving in new material, combining of new material with what is already present in memory stores in the cortex, always guided by emotion.

Emotion tells one what is important to an individual. In other words I suggest that the emotion-guided making of connections not only produces the dream image but also integrates and updates one's memory systems in the cortex.

I want to make it clear that I am not speaking of memory consolidation, a process well studied in animals, referring to the ease of recall of specific memories. It is quite possible that sleep, among its functions, does play a role in memory consolidation. The studies that have been referred to showing replay of waking patterns in hippocampal neurons during sleep may be relevant to this role.[1,2] But I suggest that dreaming, which is a form of mental functioning—basically meaning cerebral cortical functioning—probably has a function relating to integration of memory. I have referred to this as a weaving together of old and new memories, and the building of memory systems guided by emotion.

There is no direct experimental proof for this (nor of any function of dreaming), but I believe one can see this integration happening, on a clinical level, if one follows long series of dreams. One can follow it most clearly after an acute traumatic event, when one is able to obtain a long series of dreams following the event, and a series of dreams before the event also, for comparison. I have collected several long dream series of this kind. Here is what happens:

The first dreams after the trauma sometimes directly portray bits of the actual events, but usually with changes as noted.

Then the emotion (especially fear, vulnerability) often is pictured in a powerful dream such as the tidal wave dream.[6,13]

Then a whole series of combinations occur in which dreams appear to be connecting memories of the actual trauma, metaphoric pictures of the emotion, and pictures of similar past traumas or other related events that have some emotional relationship to the new one.

Finally, usually after a few months, the dreams gradually return to the pattern they had before the traumatic event.

For instance, here is a case of a definite but relatively mild trauma. A sensitive boy, 14 years old, on a trip with his parents, was inadvertently locked into a hotel room for a day and a half. Apparently, there was no phone, and no one heard him when he yelled and pounded on the doors and walls. He became extremely upset for a time before he was finally rescued. He summarized what happened over the next months:

"I then had many dreams and nightmares about this event. I was always locked in, enclosed or trapped in some way, but the dreams gradually changed. Sometimes I was trapped in a room like the actual one, sometimes in a very different situation. I also dreamt of being caught in a fire and of drowning in a tidal wave. Sometimes my parents were there; sometimes scenes from my childhood—scenes involving being caught or trapped—entered into the dreams. My dreams were playing with the theme of my being trapped in a room and bringing in all kinds of related stuff from my life, from stories I'd read and from my imaginings."

He says it took 4 or 5 months for his dreams to gradually finish dealing with the traumatic event, and to return to the themes they had before the incident.

Here is a situation involving a more severe trauma. This was a 30-year-old man who lived in Oklahoma City at the time of the Federal Building bombing in 1995. One of his friends died in the bombing.

He was a good dream recaller who wrote down his dreams and was willing to share about 200 consecutive dreams occurring before, and for a year after, the bombing. Before the date of the bombing he had a lot of dreams involving his work and his friends, and a few nightmares also. On the day of the bombing his sleep and his dreams changed drastically. For a few nights he slept poorly and could not remember dreaming at all. Then for a few days he had brief dreams of simply driving to the Federal Building and sitting there in his car. Then he had similar dreams that included his driving there and looking around, noticing that the streets were empty; he was the only one there. He saw the scene very powerfully and vividly, but nothing more happened. In one dream he drove to the building, opened his car door and got out. In one dream there were other people there, and a friend opened the car door for him. Then he had a powerful dream of a large stadium. A police helicopter dropped a man, apparently the chief suspect in the bombing, into the stadium, and the whole crowd, all 85,000 or so, went after him to kill him. Then some dreams of himself in an auditorium, feeling very uncomfortable. He was being grilled—questioned—by people up on the podium. Then he had dreams of being chased by gangsters, and especially of a friend being hurt by gangsters. There were dreams of a Ryder truck, the same kind used in the bombing, coming to his house. He additionally had dreams of storm clouds, violent whirlwinds, and many kinds of danger. He had dreams of fighting and dreams that incorporated fights and conflicts from his childhood along with recent scenes related to the bombing. Almost all the dreams had very powerful images, usually images involving danger. Many of the dreams clearly pictured his emotions, including especially terror, vulnerability, and anger.

Only very gradually, about 5 to 8 months after the bombing, did the violent themes start to subside. His dreams gradually calmed down, with more dreams of friends and girlfriends, concerns about his work, with less powerful images. All his dreams were scored for central images.[6] The intensity scores were very high in the months after the bombing, and then gradually decreased back to their prebombing levels over the subsequent year.

So, in these cases involving a single traumatic event, one can trace a gradual playing with and weaving in of new traumatic material. I suggest that this happens all the time, but is harder to follow when there is no single marker event, such as an acute trauma.

I suggest, though I cannot prove, that this connecting and combining process after trauma can be useful (adaptive) in several related ways. First of all, once these connections are made, the material is not so frightening. The dreamer no longer feels "this is the most horrible thing that has ever happened to anyone, how can I survive this?" The dreamer rather notes that this experience is "somewhat like… is not too different from…, reminds me of… " This may be useful in itself, and in addition, the connections between such traumatic events and the existing memory stores will be useful in making a new trauma less distressing if it should happen again, or if something similar should happen.

This is an example of the suggested functions of dreaming in integrating new experience into memory, guided by emotion. This structuring of one's memories along emotional lines is what makes up one's personal sense of meaning and sense of self as has been noted by a number of thinkers, for instance Rapaport[26] and Modell,[27] starting from their own frames of reference. In this sense, I suggest that dreaming plays a role in what one can call the creation of personal meaning and a sense of self.

THE CONTEMPORARY THEORY OF DREAMING

This discussion of dreaming above fits closely into what has been called the Contemporary Theory of Dreaming[15,28]:

Dreaming is a form of mental functioning. It is not an alien intrusion, not material in a foreign language, and not separable from one's other mental functioning. It is one end of a continuum of mental functioning (which means chiefly cerebral cortical functioning) running from focused waking thought at one end, through reverie, daydreaming, and fantasy to dreaming at the other end.

Dreaming is hyperconnective. At the dreaming end of the continuum, connections are made more easily than in waking, and connections are made more broadly and loosely. Dreaming avoids tightly structured, overlearned material. One does not dream of the three Rs. Dreaming always involves new connections; dreaming is creation, not replay.

The connections are not made randomly. They are guided by the emotions of the dreamer. The dream, and especially the central image of the dream, pictures or expresses the dreamer's emotion or emotional concerns. The more powerful the emotion, the more powerful (intense) is the central image.

The form or language of dreams is mainly picture–metaphor. But this is not a language restricted to dreaming. It is the way things are expressed toward the right-hand end of the continuum. At this end of the continuum there is less serial processing, less task orientation, less functioning by formal rules, less constraint. The system relaxes into a default mode, functioning by similarity (metaphor), rather than formal rules, guided by whatever emotions or emotional concerns are present.

Functions of dreaming. This making of broad connections guided by emotion has an adaptive function, which we conceptualize as weaving in new material—taking new experiences and gradually connecting them, integrating them, into existing memory systems. In other words, the dream helps one to build and rebuild a meaningful emotional memory system, which is the basis of one's individual self.

This primary function occurs regardless of whether a dream is remembered. When a dream is remembered, the broad connections also can be adaptive in increasing self-knowledge and producing new insights and creations.

Function of the continuum. In addition to the functions of dreaming, the entire focused waking-to-dreaming continuum has an adaptive function. It is obviously useful to be able to think in direct, focused, serial fashion at certain times, and at other times to associate more broadly, and loosely—in other words to daydream and to dream.

USING DREAMS IN THERAPY AND IN SELF-KNOWLEDGE

Finally, I believe that this discussion of dreams as creative products always making new connections has implications for one's use of dreams in therapy and in getting to know oneself. Based on what already has been discussed and a great deal of other work on dreaming,[14,28] I believe that no complete translation of a dream is possible. The dream is a creative part of one's mental functioning, but it is not neatly translatable into one's waking thoughts or waking language. I cannot agree with Freud's view of the dream as only a "manifest dream" that can be translated completely into a group of underlying thoughts (the "latent dream"). One indeed can work on a dream and free associate to the elements in the dream. Underlying thoughts and especially underlying emotional concerns usually emerge. Discussion of the underlying latent thoughts definitely can contribute to one's understanding, but in my view one can no more substitute the latent thoughts for the dream than one can substitute a critic's explanation of a work of art for the work of art itself.

I suggest that probably all one can usefully do is get to the gist of the dream. Getting the gist involves appreciating the dream as a whole, looking at the connections to see if there is anything new or surprising, and examining the central image to help identify the underlying emotion and concerns. Most often, that is all one can do with certainty, in terms of understanding the dream, and perhaps it is all one should do.

Of course one needs not stop there. When one has a truly impressive dream, a "big" dream, it can be so striking that it calls out for attention, although not necessarily interpretation. In fact interpretation may be the wrong approach. Interpretation emphasizes finding a meaning, a latent dream under the dream and more or less substituting that for the dream. Of course dreaming is meaningful, as is thought, fantasy, daydreaming, and artistic creation. But there is not a single meaning to be extracted. I suggest that rather than translating the dream, one can appreciate it, admire it, learn from it.

IMPORTANT POINTS

Every dream makes new connections. The dream is a creative product, not a replay of waking material. The connections in dreaming are not made randomly; they are guided by the emotions of the dreamer. Dreaming may have a function in integrating new with old memories, guided by emotion. This is very different from memory consolidation.

REFERENCES

1. Wilson MA, McNaughton BL. Reactivation of hippocampal ensemble memories during sleep. Science 1994;265:676–9.
2. Qin YL, McNaughton BL, Skaggs WE, et al. Memory reprocessing in cortico–cortical and hippocampo–cortical neuronal ensembles. Philos Trans R Soc Lond B Biol Sci 1997;352:1525–33.
3. Nielsen TA, Kuiken D, Alain G, et al. Immediate and delayed incorporations of events into dreams: further replications and implications for dream function. J Sleep Res 2004;13(4):327–36.
4. Nielsen TA, Stenstrom P. What are the memory sources of dreaming? Nature 2005;437(7063):1286–9.
5. Hartmann E. The day residue: time distribution of waking events [abstract]. Psychophysiology 1968;5:222.
6. Hartmann E, Zborowski M, Rosen R, et al. Contextualizing images in dreams: more intense after abuse and trauma. Dreaming 2001;11:115–26.
7. Hartmann E, Brezler T. A systematic change in dreams after 9/11/01. Sleep 2008;31:213–8.
8. Cartwright R, Romanek I. Repetitive dreams of normal subjects. Sleep Research 1978;7:174.
9. Robbins P, Houshi F. Some observations on recurrent dreams. Bull Menninger Clin 1983;47:262–5.
10. Domhoff WG. Finding meaning in dreams: a quantitative approach. New York: Plenum Press; 1996.
11. Hartmann E. The nightmare: the psychology and biology of terrifying dreams. New York: Basic Books; 1984.
12. American Psychiatric Association. DSM-IV-TR: diagnostic and statistical manual of mental disorders. Washington, DC: American Psychiatric Association; 2000.
13. Hartmann E. Outline for a theory on the nature and functions of dreaming. Dreaming 1996;6:147–70.
14. Hartmann E. Dreams and nightmares: the new theory on the origin and meaning of dreams. Perseus Books. New York: Plenum Press; 1998/2001.
15. Hartmann E. The nature and functions of dreaming. In: Barrett D, McNamara P, editors, The new science of dreaming, vol. 3. Westport (CT): Praeger; 2007. p. 171–92.
16. Hobson JA. The dreaming brain. New York: Basic Books; 1988.
17. Fiss H, Klein GS, Bokert E. Waking fantasies following interruption of two types of sleep. Arch Gen Psychiatry 1966;14:543–51.
18. Stickgold R, Scott L, Rittenhouse C, et al. Sleep induced changes in associative memory. J Cogn Neurosci 1999;11:182–93.
19. Hartmann E. We do not dream of the 3 R's: implications for the nature of dreaming mentation. Dreaming 2000;10:103–11.
20. Hartmann E. The psychology and physiology of dreaming: a new synthesis. In: Gamwell L, editor. Dreams 1900–2000: science, art, and the unconscious mind. New York: State University of New York Press; 1999. p. 61–76.
21. Stevenson RL. Across the plains. Leipzig (Germany): Bernhard Tauchnitz; 1892.
22. Eliot TS. Prufrock and other observations. London: Egoist Press; 1917.
23. Barrett D. The committee of sleep. New York: Crown Publishers; 2001.
24. Foulkes D. Children's dreams. New York: Wiley; 1982.
25. Foulkes D. Children's dreaming and the development of consciousness. Cambridge (MA): Harvard University Press; 1999.
26. Rapaport D. The conceptual model of psychoanalysis. In: Krech D, Klein GS, editors. Theoretical models and personality theory. Durham (NC): Duke University Press; 1952. p. 56–81.
27. Modell A. Imagination and the meaningful brain. Cambridge (MA): MIT Press; 2003.
28. Hartmann E. The nature and functions of dreaming. New York: Oxford University Press; 2010, in press.

Frequency and Content of Dreams Associated with Trauma

Mylène Duval, PhD(c)[a], Antonio Zadra, PhD[b],*

KEYWORDS

- Dreaming • Dream frequency • Dream content
- Nightmares • Trauma • Posttraumatic dreams

According to the Diagnostic and statistical manual of mental disorders, fourth edition—text revision (DSM-IV-TR),[1] traumatic events can occur when an individual experiences or witnesses an event that involves a threat to the integrity of self or others, accompanied by intense fear, helplessness, or horror. Rape, physical assaults, war exposure, severe automobile accidents, the sudden unexpected death of a loved one, and natural disasters constitute examples of traumatic experiences. Depending on how traumatic events are defined, epidemiologic studies indicate that the lifetime prevalence of exposure to at least one traumatic event in the general population ranges from more than 50% to almost 90%.[2–4] Exposure to such events can lead to a variety of physical, behavioral, emotional, and cognitive sequelae, and a small but significant subset of trauma victims (fewer than 10%) will develop posttraumatic stress disorder (PTSD).[3–5]

Sleep disturbances and dream-related disorders are some of the most frequently reported and persistent symptoms shown by trauma victims,[6–8] and nightmares have been described as a hallmark of PTSD.[9–11] Recurrent distressing trauma-related dreams are one of the ways an individual may reexperience a traumatic event, and they are considered a core symptom of PTSD (Cluster B) in the DSM-IV-TR manual.

The prominent role of sleep disturbances and dream-related disorders in trauma victims' clinical profiles has been highlighted in research on survivors of abuse and sexual trauma,[12–14] natural disasters,[15–18] war victims or veterans,[19,20] and victims or witnesses of sudden deaths, violent acts, and accidents.[21–23]

Although there has been a growing interest in the role of sleep mechanisms and nightmares in the development, maintenance, and treatment of PTSD,[24–27] little is known about the actual content of trauma-related dreams and nightmares associated with PTSD and with trauma in general. In their recent review of dreaming in PTSD, Wittmann and colleagues[24] concluded that "we have alarmingly little reliable information characterizing the phenomenology of the disturbing dream in PTSD" (page 36). Moreover, little effort has been made to integrate empirical and clinical findings on the dreams of trauma victims that do not necessarily meet the diagnostic criteria for PTSD.

This article reviews and synthesizes findings on the frequency and content of trauma-related dreams, beyond the boundaries of posttraumatic nightmares associated with PTSD. Methodological issues that complicate data comparisons across studies are examined. Findings on dream recall frequency following trauma exposure are reviewed and factors believed to impact dream

This work was supported by a grant from the Social Sciences and Humanities Research Council of Canada (SSHRC).

[a] Surgery/Traumatology Unit, Centre Hospitalier Universitaire Sainte Justine, Montreal, QC, Canada
[b] Department of Psychology, Université de Montréal, CP 6128, Succursale Centre-ville, Montreal, QC H3C 3J7, Canada
* Corresponding author.
E-mail address: antonio.zadra@umontreal.ca

Sleep Med Clin 5 (2010) 249–260
doi:10.1016/j.jsmc.2010.01.003

recall over time are highlighted. The incidence of dream-related disorders is then examined as a function of trauma characteristics and personality variables. Findings on the relationship between dream content and specific types of traumas are subsequently reviewed. Finally, the clinical importance of furthering the knowledge of dream-related disorders in trauma victims is discussed.

METHODOLOGICAL ISSUES
Terminology

A wide range of phenotypic and phenomenological expressions and disagreements exist among researchers and clinicians on the concepts and nosologic terms best suited to describe and categorize trauma-related dreams. Similarly, differing views exist on how traumatic experiences as well as trauma severity are defined. Regarding sleep mentation, there is no consensus on how dreams should be defined, and there exist important discrepancies and variations in how nightmares are operationalized in both clinical and research settings.[26]

Schreuder and colleagues[28] proposed a classification system to distinguish between a range of dream experiences, including those related to trauma (**Table 1**), but this system has rarely been used. However, Schreuder and colleagues' definition of a nightmare is consistent with DSM-IV-TR criteria for nightmare disorder, and their use of the term "anxiety dream" corresponds to what some investigators commonly refer to as bad dreams.[29] Taking a different approach and based

on their comprehensive and integrative conceptual framework, Levin and Nielsen[26] proposed a typology of dreaming, ranging from normal dreaming to replicative posttraumatic nightmares, which is organized by increasing affect load (ie, fluctuations in current levels of affect), affect distress (ie, a disposition to experience events with distressing, highly reactive emotions), and trauma severity (**Fig. 1**). As in Schreuder and colleagues' classification, awakenings from sleep distinguish dysphoric and bad dreaming from nightmares. Although such developments are conceptually valuable and promising, only their wider adoption will allow for an increasingly unified and more easily comparable framework across studies.

Frequency Measurement

Traditionally, nightmare frequency has been assessed with retrospective questionnaires that require participants to estimate the number of nightmares experienced in the past, usually using binary, nominal, ordinal, or open-ended choices. When compared with daily logs, however, retrospective self-reports significantly underestimate nightmare frequency.[29,30] Prospective daily logs have supplanted retrospective questionnaires as the gold standard for nightmare frequency estimation, but this method of data collection is not always used owing to costs and time requirements. Recent findings[31] indicate that prospective studies of dream recall and nightmare frequency should take the type of log used (ie, narrative form or

Table 1	
Classification and definition of dreams and nightmares	
Dream Type	**Definition**
Dream	Reportable mental activity that occurs during sleep
Anxiety dream	Frightening dream that does not awaken the dreamer but recalled only after waking up in the morning
Nightmare	Frightening dream that awakens the sleeper
Posttraumatic dream	Dream content is associated with traumatic events by the dreamer
Posttraumatic anxiety dream	Frightening posttraumatic dream recalled only after waking up in the morning
Posttraumatic nightmare	Frightening posttraumatic dream that awakens the sleeper
Replicative posttraumatic nightmare	Dream content is a replication of the original traumatic event
Nonreplicative or symbolic posttraumatic nightmare	Dream content can be trauma-related but not a replay of the traumatic event

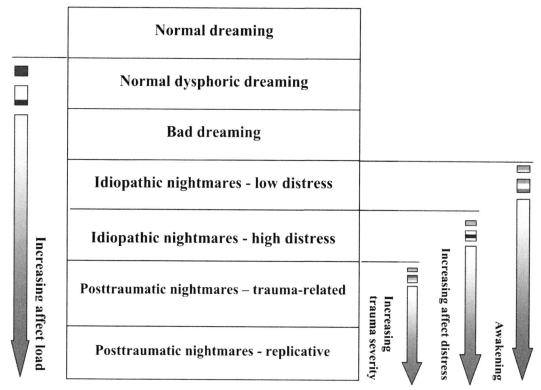

Fig. 1. Typology of dreaming organized by increasing affect load, affect distress, and trauma severity. Normal dreaming, dysphoric dreaming, bad dreaming, and idiopathic nightmares with low distress are all considered to be nonpathological in that trauma precursors are absent and participants report low levels of associated distress. Awakenings from sleep distinguish dysphoric and bad dreaming from idiopathic nightmares with low distress. Idiopathic nightmares with high distress, posttraumatic trauma-related nightmares, and posttraumatic replicative nightmares are all considered pathologic because of the subjective affect distress associated with them. Posttraumatic nightmares produce even more distress in step with the number and severity of trauma precursors. (*From* Levin R, Nielsen TA. Disturbed dreaming, posttraumatic stress disorder, and affect distress: a review and neurocognitive model. Psychol Bull 2007;133(3):482–528; with permission.)

simple checklist), its duration, and the participants' level of motivation over time into account, because these factors can influence the log-based reporting of dreams and nightmares. Finally, regarding trauma-related nightmares, the amount of time elapsed between the occurrence of a traumatic event and the assessment of nightmares potentially associated to the event is an important variable that is not always taken into account or even explicitly reported in research and clinical articles.

TRAUMA AND DREAM RECALL FREQUENCY

Increases in dream recall have been reported in normal individuals facing a stressful situation,[32] and analogous findings have been found in people exposed to traumatic events.[19,33,34] In a study of children exposed to war, Valli and colleagues[34] found that severely traumatized children reported a significantly greater number of dreams when compared with less traumatized or nontraumatized children. Investigating a similar population, Helminen and Punamaki[19] found that Palestinian children living under conditions of military violence and war in Gaza reported a greater number of dreams than children living in the more peaceful areas of Galilee. Within this study's trauma group, the number of dreams reported was greater in children exposed to higher levels of trauma. Taken together, these studies indicate that increased dream recall frequency is positively associated to trauma severity or to more direct exposure to a traumatic event. Dream recall may also be facilitated by the intensity, affective charge, and references to the victims' trauma as depicted in their dreams.[11,34–36]

Other studies, however, report a significant reduction in dream recall following exposure to stressful situations,[6,7,37–39] but these findings are largely based on retrospective assessments conducted months, or even years, following trauma exposure. It is possible that dream recall increases immediately following exposure to trauma and diminishes subsequently over time.

A comparison[39] of well-adjusted Holocaust survivors, less-adjusted Holocaust survivors, and controls found that the well-adjusted survivors reported fewer dreams from rapid eye movement (REM) sleep (33.7%) compared with the less-adjusted survivors (50.5%) and controls (80.8%). A reduction in dream recall may thus reflect improved posttrauma adaptation.

Finally, sleep laboratory investigations of patients suffering from PTSD[40–42] suggest that disruption of REM sleep—as indicated by increased sleep stage transitions, awakening threshold and arousal, and increased symptho-vagal tone—is associated with increased PTSD symptom severity and may increase the likelihood of developing PTSD at follow-up assessments. Thus, REM sleep disruption and increased arousal during REM sleep may amplify one's vulnerability to experience more vivid and hostile dreams following trauma exposure and to develop PTSD.

TRAUMA AND DREAM-RELATED DISTURBANCES

Exposure to traumatic events can give rise to a range of dream-related disturbances, including a higher prevalence of posttraumatic dreams, nightmares, bad dreams, and recurrent dreams. The emergence and frequency of such dream-related disturbances can be mediated by characteristics associated with the traumatic event itself as well as to the individual exposed to it. These variables are reviewed in turn.

Trauma-Related Variables

Observed differences across studies investigating the frequency of dream-related disorders in trauma victims seem to be caused by, at least in part, variations in the trauma's severity, the degree of exposure to the event, and to the amount of time elapsed between the investigation and the trauma's original occurrence.

In a study of 598 female victims of sexual assault, Krakow and colleagues[43] found that the degree of severity of the trauma was associated with nightmare frequency. Specifically, women who reported suffering the most severe sexual aggressions were the most likely to report experiencing frequent nightmares.

Similarly, the degree of exposure to the trauma is another important factor affecting the experience of distressing dreams. Among the children who were victims of a school shooting, 63% of those who were in the school yard directly at the scene of the shooting reported experiencing bad dreams, compared with 56% of the children who were inside the school, 43% of those who were not at school (eg, at home), and 33% of those who were not in the geographic area where the shooting occurred (eg, away on holidays).[44] Comparable results were found by Wood and colleagues,[17] who collected prospective measures of dream recall (including nightmares) from college students for 3 weeks following the Loma Prieta earthquake. Results showed that the students who witnessed direct impacts of the earthquake (eg, injuries, material losses, imminent threats) reported twice as many nightmares than college students living in a nearby state.

A positive relationship between frequency of dreams with threatening themes and degree of trauma exposure was also found in investigations of more chronic traumatic environments. In their study of victims of war, Valli and colleagues[34] found that 80% of Kurdish children directly exposed to armed conflict reported experiencing threatening dreams in a 1-week dream journal, compared with 56% of children living in a more peaceful zone of the same region and 31% of children not exposed to war.

Although dream-related disorders can persist for varying periods of time following trauma exposure, the amount of time elapsed since the traumatic event's occurrence can also impact their duration and frequency. One study[45] of rape victims found an increased rate of nightmares (31%) immediately after the trauma, in comparison with a decrease of 21% 1 year after the event. Terr's[46,47] longitudinal investigations of a group of children who had been kidnapped revealed that 96% of them were still experiencing repeated terror dreams 4 years after the kidnapping. A reduction in nightmare frequency in people exposed to an earthquake was similarly obtained by Wood and colleagues[17] in the weeks following the earthquake.

Although trauma victims tend to experience a reduction in nightmares and other forms of distressing dreams after the acute phase of trauma exposure, dream disturbances can persist for years or even decades, sometimes with little to no change in their content.[48]

Individual-Related Variables

Following trauma exposure, individual-related variables including psychological reaction to trauma (eg, level of anxiety, distress), psychopathology, and personality characteristics can sometimes play a key role in determining the frequency of dream-related disorders.

The impact of individual psychological reactions during the acute phase of trauma on the frequency of dream-related disorders was investigated in several studies. Wood and colleagues[17] showed that people's nightmare frequencies following an earthquake were related to the individuals' assessments of their anxiety levels during the event but not to the earthquake's objective level of danger (eg, risk of death or serious injury) nor to the individuals' general levels of anxiety as retrospectively estimated for the 24 hours preceding the event.

The initial psychological response (including the occurrence of nightmares) experienced by some people in reaction to a traumatic event can persist over time and affect the frequency of dream-related disorders while contributing to the development of psychopathology. Mellmann and colleagues[49] found that the victims of Hurricane Andrew who went on to develop PTSD reported a higher frequency of bad dreams than the victims who did not develop it. Similarly, a study[50] of patients reporting posttraumatic symptoms revealed that individuals who suffered from chronic nightmares experienced higher levels of depression, anxiety, and posttraumatic stress. Furthermore, in their investigation of control subjects and sexually abused women 10 years after disclosure of the substantiated abuse, Noll and colleagues[14] showed that after taking the levels of comorbid psychopathology (eg, depression, PTSD) into account, sexually abused women reported significantly greater rates of sleep disturbances, including nightmares, than did the control participants.

TRAUMA AND DREAM CONTENT
Trauma Replication and Repetition in Dreams

Trauma-related dreams may depict a replication of the traumatic event, its modified versions, or metaphorical representations that may evolve over time. However, various terms have been used to describe such dream experiences, and no consensus exists on how best to categorize them. Two dream-related indicators of the severity of a trauma's impact on the victim stand out in the literature, namely, the traumatic replication, which refers to the similarities between posttrauma dream content and the actual traumatic event,[11,20,26,46] and the traumatic repetition, which refers to the recurrence of the traumatic dream imagery.[11,46] Both indicators exist on a continuum. Because some traumatic dreams may contain a high level of distress, sometimes in the absence of actual trauma-related imagery, Levin and Nielsen[26] also suggest the use of a continuum for distress related to traumatic dreams. Whether or not the dreamer awakens from the disturbing dream can also be used as a criterion for differentiating nightmares from bad dreams that contain traumatic elements.[26,28]

Dreams that, to varying extents, replicate traumatic events have been documented in various populations including war veterans,[20,42,51] people exposed to war,[39] child witnesses of violence and abuse,[44,47,52,53] burn victims,[54] individuals exposed to natural disasters,[16,17] and more recently, in US residents following the 9/11 terrorist attacks.[55]

Trauma victims can report both exact and modified replicas of the traumatic event in their dreams.[47,51,53,56] In a study[56] of 316 Vietnam War veterans, 304 veterans reported combat-related nightmares. An examination of their dream narratives showed that more than 50% of the veterans reported realistic combat dreams, 21% reported plausible war sequences that they nevertheless had not experienced, and 26% reported dreams that alluded to the war but included fantastical and everyday elements among others. In addition, a laboratory study of war veterans found that only 21% of dreams exactly replicate the traumatic event whereas 79% contain distortions of the traumatic event.[51] Similarly, a study[21] of patients hospitalized following an accident or assault found that 48% of the reported dreams replicated the traumatic event, of these, 33% were dissimilar to the traumatic event while containing high levels of distress. Finally, a study of battered women[57] found modified memories of the abuse in the women's dreams but none that exactly replicated the trauma.

Trauma victims may also experience nightmares whose contents do not show direct links or references to the original trauma.[47,57,58] Waiess,[57] for instance, noted several spontaneous reports of nightmares or "symbolic or metaphoric" dreams among battered women who described these particular dreams as having the same terror quality as that experienced when facing their aggressor, although the dream's content was not linked to the actual event. These results suggest that although the nonaffective content of such dreams may not show any clear relations to the original trauma, they may nevertheless contain significant trauma-related emotional distress.

Finally, Hartmann's[11,59] clinical investigations of dream series collected from patients immediately after their exposure to trauma as well as afterward indicate that dreams recalled soon after a traumatic experience generally contain direct references to the actual event, although only a minority of the dreams depict exact replicas of the trauma. The dreams' contents then change progressively over time, becoming dissimilar to the actual event while dealing more exclusively with contextualizing images associated with a succession of traumatic emotions, including fear, guilt, and grief. Although the PTSD status of these patients is not reported, this pattern is consistent with other findings highlighting the central role of traumatic or intense emotions related to trauma in dream imagery following a traumatic event.

Heightened exposure to trauma can also augment the likelihood of intrusion of trauma-related memories into dream imagery, as shown in children exposed to a school shooting,[44] victims of an earthquake,[17] and former combatants and individuals exposed to war.[20,60] More severe, intense, and directly experienced stressors thus seem to give rise to greater levels of intrusion of traumatic images in victims' dreams.

Intrusion of traumatic imagery in victims' dreams may reflect or contribute to difficulties with posttraumatic adaptation and psychological adjustment. One study[39] of Holocaust survivors showed that those whose dreams contained direct references to the Holocaust had lowered postwar levels of adaptation. Similar results have been reported in other populations diagnosed with PTSD.[15,42,61] For example, Mellman and colleagues[42] found that 65% of veterans suffering from PTSD reported nightmares of combat at least once a week, compared with only 5% of veterans without PTSD.

Taken together, these findings indicate that traumatic dreams with realistic trauma scenes are not present among all trauma victims, and that the intrusion of an exact replica of a traumatic event in dreams is generally not a frequent or long-lasting phenomenon. The acute phase associated with severe trauma tends to be accompanied by higher levels of posttraumatic dreams replicating the trauma, although the frequency of these dreams subsequently diminishes over time.[46,47,53,55] Dreams that initially include some degree of replication of an experienced trauma also tend to be followed by dreams more likely to contain symbolic representations or distortions of the trauma as well as references to the dreamer's daily waking life. These changes in dream content can parallel improvements in the posttrauma reaction[39,61,62] and thus may serve as indicators of clinical progress in trauma victims' responses to trauma.

Dreamlike Versus Ordinary Quality of Dream Content

Findings from studies in younger populations suggest that when compared with the dream reports from controls, dreams recalled by trauma victims tend to be more ordinary and realistic and less salient, bizarre, and imaginative. For instance, a lack of so-called dreamlike qualities (referring to properties associated with daydreaming, imagination, and distortion) has been observed in the dreams of children living in violent environments.[33,63,64] A more direct and chronic exposure to violent environments is related to more realistic or ordinary dreams in children.[63] It is not clear, however, if such differences in the dreamlike quality of dream reports are maintained over time. Studies of adult students reporting a history of childhood abuse reveal no differences in the length or the dreamlike quality of dream reports provided by victims of abuse versus controls.[36]

Turning to trauma-exposed adults, although one study[35] of a dream series collected from US residents (not from New York) both before and after the 9/11 terrorist attacks found no differences in their levels of intensity and bizarreness, another study[55] focusing on students living in the New York area found that the sooner after the 9/11 attacks a dream was collected, the more intense and bizarre it tended to be. In their investigation of Holocaust survivors, Lavie and Kaminer[38] found that the dreams of less-adjusted survivors contained similar features to those from nontraumatized controls, whereas well-adjusted survivors had shorter, less complex, more imaginative, vivid, and salient dreams.

All these findings suggest that the "ordinary" quality of trauma victims' dreams may reflect an alteration in the process of dream construction or may be related to a protective mechanism that keeps traumatic images from intruding into their everyday dreams. Ordinary or realistic aspects of survivors' dreams may thus be associated with more adaptive ways of coping with trauma,[37,38,63] although increases in the dreamlike quality of survivors' dreams can occur with the passage of time.

Emotions

Emotions are viewed by many dream theorists as a key player in structuring dream content.[65] Hartmann and colleagues[11,59,66] proposed a model suggesting that dreams may regulate emotions by contextualizing the dreamer's primary emotional concern or dominant emotion in a central image (eg, a tidal wave). In addition, the intensity of trauma-related emotions may be represented by the dream's central image's strength or power. In line with the model's predictions, one controlled study[36] found that dreams of abused victims contained more intense central images than the dreams of control participants. Similarly, one investigation of people's dreams before and after the 9/11 terrorists attacks found that the emotional intensity of the dreams' central images increased after 9/11.[67]

The representation of emotional intensity in dreams' central images was also investigated in children exposed to traumatic events. In a study of dream reports from Palestinian children living in a militarized area, 90% of the dreams were found to contain a central image that contextualized an emotion, whereas such central images occurred in only 74% of dream reports provided by children living in a more peaceful region.[19] The dreams of children exposed to war were more likely to incorporate more intense and negative emotional images than the dreams of children without trauma exposure.

Several studies have observed that the dreams of trauma victims often contain trauma-related dysphoric emotions, thereby suggesting continuity between waking emotional states and the valence of emotions experienced in dreams. For example, children exposed to multiple traumatic events within the environmental context of war report more negative valence in their dreams' emotional images than children exposed to less severe traumas.[19] Children experiencing traumatic events are also more likely to report feelings of anxiety and hostility in their dreams.[63,68] Similarly, clinical and empirical reports indicate that victims of sexual abuse or aggression tend to report emotions of fear, terror, sadness, and helplessness in their dreams and nightmares,[69–71] whereas emotional themes involving anxiety, hostility, guilt, and persecution have been documented in the dreams of Holocaust survivors.[37] These findings suggest that the emotional content of trauma victims' dreams can be related to the emotional reaction to their traumatic event.[72]

Finally, there is evidence to suggest that emotional preoccupations before bedtime may also play a role in the affective content experienced during subsequent sleep. One study[33] of 413 dream journals collected from Palestinian children exposed to chronic conditions of war showed that going to sleep in a negative mood (eg, scared, angry, worried) was associated with positive dreams, whereas going to sleep in a good mood was associated with dysphoric dreams. The finding that one's mood prior to sleep is inversely related to a positive or negative dream affect supports the idea that dreams may have a restorative function by helping regulate emotional equilibrium in traumatized individuals.[11,73] It is also possible that dream-mediated processes of trauma integration protect individuals from overwhelming intrusions of traumatic imagery into their dreams,[64] whereas a disturbance dream's restorative function could account for the occurrence of replicative nightmares associated with high levels of psychological distress.

RELATIONSHIP BETWEEN DREAM CONTENT AND SPECIFIC TYPES OF TRAUMAS

A few studies have focused attention on identifying specific features of dream content in relation to specific types of traumas, notably in combatants and victims of natural disasters, physical and sexual abuse, and war and violence. This literature, beyond being of interest in itself, might also help to clarify how trauma is possibly integrated into dreams.

Victims of Physical and Sexual Abuse

Abuse, whether physical or sexual, always involves a threat to the individual's physical and psychological integrity. Not surprisingly, dreams of victims of abuse can contain high proportions of violent themes.[13,69–72,74] For example, themes of attack and pursuit are more often reported by victims of sexual abuse than by control participants,[52,69,70,74] and themes of being threatened, directly confronting an attacker, or obtaining revenge have been reported in dreams of children having witnessed their mother's rape.[52]

Although themes of violence and aggression are ubiquitous in people's dreams, empirical investigations reveal increased levels of physical aggression in the dreams of female victims of abuse.[70,71] Fernandez and colleagues[75] found more episodes of verbal and physical abuse in the dreams of physically abused women (88% verbal; 75% physical) as compared with the dreams of a control group (25% verbal; 33% physical). Dreaming about one's own death is also more frequent in sexually abused women than in control participants,[69–71,74,75] and victims of sexual abuse are more likely to report nightmares that include blood and dismemberment.[13,71,76]

In addition, dreams of victims of sexual abuse are more likely to contain references to negative sexual activity[69–72,77] while their nightmares are characterized by increased frequencies of negative sexual themes including lack of trust, shame, guilt, jealousy, anger, and violence.[13,70,71] In addition, one study[77] of female victims of rape, incest, or sexual abuse found that their dreams contained themes of aggression and sexuality where the sexuality was unpredictable and resulted in fear.

There is also evidence indicating that characters represent a distinguishing dimension in abused women's dreams. Nightmares reported by sexually abused women are more likely to contain unknown male characters, sometimes depicted as being faceless or more like shadows or demons, than nightmares of nonabused women.[13,71,76] Abused women are also more likely than nonabused women to report feeling a "presence" in their dreams.[13,70,71,76] Victims of sexual abuse have also been described as reporting the presence of serpents or worms, and these references are more frequently found in the dreams of sexually abused women than in those of physically abused women.[12] References in abused women's dreams to both sexual and nonsexual body parts have also been noted.[12,69] Finally, one study of battered and nonbattered women[57] revealed that unpleasant dreams about husbands represented 4% of the total number of dreams recorded by the nonbattered women but 14% of that recorded by the battered women. By contrast, unpleasant or violent dreams about husbands were as infrequent in the dream records of the nonbattered women as pleasant dreams about the batterers were infrequent in the dream records of the battered women.

Combatants and Victims of War and Violence

War trauma constitutes a serious risk factor in the development and increase of posttraumatic depressive and anxiety symptoms.[78] Valli and colleagues[34] showed that when compared with children living in a peaceful area, children exposed to war report a greater number of threatening events per dream and a higher percentage of dreams that include a threat. Exposure to an environment of war or violence is also associated with dreams depicting increased aggressive and hostile human interactions.[33,37,64,68] The study of Holocaust survivors by Kaminer and Lavie[37] revealed that dreamed aggression was often self-directed in the dreams of the survivors, whereas it was usually directed toward others in the dreams from controls. Finally, Bilu[68] observed that the dreams of Arab and Israeli children represent the conflict and negative interactions between these two populations and often contain various manifestations of violence and aggression.

Victims of violence have more dreams with anxious content compared with a control group, including themes involving danger to one's own life, being physically attacked, or attempts to escape to save one's life.[39] Some war veterans also report that their traumatic dreams often entail being killed in the place of their compatriots.[61] In a study of children by Valli and colleagues,[34] the self was the most often threatened person in the dreams of both the traumatized and the control group, but the threats to the self reported by the trauma group were more dangerous (eg, death of self or parents, severe injury to self). More than half of the threats reported by the Finnish children were everyday misfortunes, rather trivial for the dream self, whereas the trauma and control groups reported life-threatening and socially, psychologically, or financially severe threats much more frequently. Similarly, a study[33] on war-exposed Palestinian children found that traumatized children had more dreams involving threatening strangers. Their dreams often comprised attacks, anxiety, persecution, hostility, and nondesirable endings. In addition, nontraumatized children reported more dreams of school and their peers than did traumatized children.[33,64] Exposure to trauma may thus increase the severity of threatening events in victims' dreams.[34]

Conflicting results have also been reported. For example, Punamäki[33] found that in addition to reporting more dreams of threatening strangers, victims of violence had more dreams referring to their family, house, affiliation, and human connections than did control participants. One study[79] of Israeli children exposed to either war or peaceful conditions found more frequent manifestations of anxiety, stress, and aggression in the dreams of children living in a peaceful climate. The finding that one's mood before sleep is inversely related to a positive or negative quality of dream content[33,64] suggests that dreams may have the function of restoring an emotional equilibrium to traumatized individuals.[11,73]

Victims of Natural Disasters

A natural disaster is an unpredictable event that generally impacts a large number of individuals. Its repercussions are noteworthy on personal, social, and economic levels. The environment that provides people with a habitat suddenly becomes a threat and a risk to one's life and physical integrity.

One investigation of victims of the East Bay Firestorm (San Francisco Bay)[16] distinguished between the dreams of 2 groups differentially affected by a forest fire that destroyed their neighborhood. Fire survivors (who lost their home and commodities) reported more dreams with general themes of loss, finding valuables, and events out of their control, as opposed to fire evacuees (who lived in the burn zone but whose homes were not destroyed by the fire), who reported more dreams with specific themes of loss and grief.

Themes of loss, grief, death, and dying were also more frequently found in the dreams of both groups than among controls. The most salient subthemes in the fire evacuees' dreams were their own deaths, the presence of someone who died, or the presence of someone actually alive who appeared dead in their dream. Both survivors' and evacuees' dreams had themes of dead animals as opposed to individuals in the control group.

Natural disasters were also more frequent in survivors' and evacuees' dreams than in the control group. Specific images included damage caused by heat and fire, floods, earthquakes, and other calamities. Fire victims also had dreams of searching for essential commodities (ie, food, clothing, and roof) and dreams regarding financial difficulties.

ARE POSTTRAUMA DREAMS ADAPTIVE?

Many contemporary dream theorists suggest that dreaming is functionally significant and may subserve a biologically important function, especially in emotional adaptation.[26,59,80] There is considerable evidence indicating that REM sleep benefits emotional processing and emotional memory consolidation[81] and that dreaming occurs preferentially during REM sleep. Regarding trauma-related dreams and nightmares, dreaming may serve as a function of emotional adaptation to emotionally salient and traumatic events. For instance, Stickgold[82] proposed a REM sleep model of the neurobiological substrates potentially subserving emotional processing and integration of trauma-related memories. Central to the model is the idea that REM sleep provides a unique neurochemical and neurobiological brain state that allows the transfer of hippocampally mediated episodic traumatic memories and amygdala-dependent salient affect into cortically distributed semantic networks.

More recently, Levin and Nielsen[26,83] proposed a comprehensive neurocognitive model of nightmare production (including bad dreams, idiopathic nightmares, and posttraumatic nightmares) emphasizing the adaptive function of fear memory extinction during dreaming. Their affect network dysfunction model, grounded on the neurophysiological roles of the amygdala, medial prefrontal cortex, hippocampus, and anterior cingulate cortex, posits that fear extinction memories can be created or maintained during dreaming via 3 key imagery processes, namely, memory element activation, memory element recombination, and emotional activation. Variations in the expression and evolution of trauma-related dreams reviewed in this article may reflect differential activations of these imagery processes and their underlying neural correlates.

Although dreaming and REM sleep may play an important role in emotional adaptation and memory integration, trauma-related dysphoric dreams and nightmares that persist over time and continue to generate distress, including in individuals who develop PTSD, may reflect a failure of these mechanisms. The repeated recall of trauma-related nightmares that awaken the sleeper (and thus do not allow habituation to physiologic arousal elicited by these memories) exposes victims to their past trauma, and may even induce retraumatization and sensitize them to trauma memories.

This literature review reveals that the systematic investigation of the content, evolution, and correlates of trauma-related dreams can give rise to a wealth of information of interest to clinicians and researchers alike. However, the paucity of research on the categorical or dimensional interrelations between various types of trauma-related dreams[26,28] and with normal dreaming severely limits our conceptual and empirical understanding of their roles and underlying processes. Similarly, much work remains to be done to clarify which specific dimensions of posttrauma sequelae and waking life functioning are most robustly associated to which kind of dream content, and the nature of these relationships over time. Recently proposed multilevel models of dysphoric dreaming[26,83] based on the integration of clinical and neurophysiological findings are promising, and represent an important step toward achieving these goals.

REFERENCES

1. American Psychiatric Association. Diagnostic and statistical manual of mental disorders, fourth edition—text revision. Washington, DC: American Psychiatric Association, Inc; 2000.
2. De Vries G-J, Olff M. The lifetime prevalence of traumatic events and posttraumatic stress disorder in the Netherlands. J Trauma Stress 2009;22(4):259–67.
3. Breslau N. The epidemiology of trauma, PTSD, and other posttrauma disorders. Trauma Violence Abuse 2009;10(3):198–210.
4. Johnson J, Maxwell A, Galea S. The epidemiology of posttraumatic stress disorder. Psychiatr Ann 2009; 39(6):326–34.
5. Kessler RC, Berglund P, Demler O, et al. Lifetime prevalence and age-of-onset distributions of DSM-IV disorders in the National Comorbidity Survey Replication. Arch Gen Psychiatry 2005;62(6):593–602.
6. Hefez A, Metz L, Lavie P. Long-term effects of extreme situational stress on sleep and dreaming. Am J Psychiatry 1987;144(3):344–7.

7. Kramer M, Kinney L. Sleep patterns in trauma victims with disturbed dreaming. Psychiatr J Univ Ott 1988;13(1):12–6.

8. Kramer M, Schoen LS, Kinney L. The dream experience in dream disturbed Vietnam veterans. In: van der Kolk BA, editor. Post-traumatic stress disorder: psychological and biological sequelae. Washington, DC: American Psychiatric Press; 1984. p. 81–95.

9. Ross RJ, Ball WA, Sullivan KA, et al. Sleep disturbance as the hallmark of posttraumatic stress disorder. Am J Psychiatry 1989;146(6):697–707.

10. Spoormaker VI, Montgomery P. Disturbed sleep in post-traumatic stress disorder: secondary symptom or core feature? Sleep Med Rev 2008;12(3):169–84.

11. Hartmann E. Nightmare after trauma as paradigm for all dreams: a new approach to the nature and functions of dreaming. Psychiatry 1998;61(3): 223–38.

12. Belicki K, Cuddy M. Identifying sexual trauma histories from patterns of sleep and dreams. In: Barrett D, editor. Trauma and dreams. Cambridge (MA): Harvard University Press; 1996. p. 46–55.

13. Cuddy MA, Belicki K. Nightmare frequency and related sleep disturbance as indicators of a history of sexual abuse. Dreaming 1992;2(1):15–22.

14. Noll JG, Trickett PK, Susman EJ, et al. Sleep disturbances and childhood sexual abuse. J Pediatr Psychol 2006;31(5):469–80.

15. David D, Mellman TA. Dreams following Hurricane Andrew. Dreaming 1997;7(3):209–14.

16. Siegel A. Dreams of firestorm survivors. In: Barrett D, editor. Trauma and dreams. Cambridge (MA): Harvard University Press; 1996. p. 159–76.

17. Wood JM, Bootzin RR, Rosenhan D, et al. Effects of the 1989 San Francisco earthquake on frequency and content of nightmares. J Abnorm Psychol 1992;101(2):219–24.

18. Najam N, Mansoor A, Kanwal RH, et al. Dream content: reflections of the emotional and psychological states of earthquake survivors. Dreaming 2006; 16(4):237–45.

19. Helminen E, Punamaki R-L. Contextualised emotional images in children's dreams: psychological adjustment in conditions of military trauma. Int J Behav Dev 2008;32(3):177–87.

20. Schreuder BJ, Kleijn WC, Rooijmans HG. Nocturnal re-experiencing more than forty years after war trauma. J Trauma Stress 2000;13(3):453–63.

21. Mellman TA, David D, Bustamante V, et al. Dreams in the acute aftermath of trauma and their relationship to PTSD. J Trauma Stress 2001;14(1):241–7.

22. Kobayashi I, Sledjeski EM, Spoonster E, et al. Effects of early nightmares on the development of sleep disturbances in motor vehicle accident victims. J Trauma Stress 2008;21(6):548–55.

23. Nielsen TA, Stenstrom P, Levin R. Nightmare frequency as a function of age, gender, and September 11, 2001: findings from an internet questionnaire. Dreaming 2006;16(3):145–58.

24. Wittmann L, Schredl M, Kramer M. Dreaming in posttraumatic stress disorder: a critical review of phenomenology, psychophysiology and treatment. Psychother Psychosom 2007;76(1):25–39.

25. Phelps AJ, Forbes D, Creamer M. Understanding posttraumatic nightmares: an empirical and conceptual review. Clin Psychol Rev 2008;28(2): 338–55.

26. Levin R, Nielsen TA. Disturbed dreaming, posttraumatic stress disorder, and affect distress: a review and neurocognitive model. Psychol Bull 2007; 133(3):482–528.

27. Germain A, Buysse DJ, Nofzinger E. Sleep-specific mechanisms underlying posttraumatic stress disorder: integrative review and neurobiological hypotheses. Sleep Med Rev 2008;12(3):185–95.

28. Schreuder BJN, Igreja V, van Dijk J, et al. Intrusive re-experiencing of chronic strife or war. Adv Psychiatr Treat 2001;7:102–8.

29. Zadra A, Donderi DC. Nightmares and bad dreams: their prevalence and relationship to well-being. J Abnorm Psychol 2000;109(2):273–81.

30. Wood JM, Bootzin RR. The prevalence of nightmares and their independence from anxiety. J Abnorm Psychol 1990;99(1):64–8.

31. Robert G, Zadra A. Measuring nightmare and bad dream frequency: impact of retrospective and prospective instruments. J Sleep Res 2008;17(2): 132–9.

32. Duke T, Davidson J. Ordinary and recurrent dream recall of active, past and non-recurrent dreamers during and after academic stress. Dreaming 2002; 12(4):185–97.

33. Punamaki R-L. The relationship of dream content and changes in daytime mood in traumatized vs. non-traumatized children. Dreaming 1999;9(4): 213–33.

34. Valli K, Revonsuo A, Palkas O, et al. The threat simulation theory of the evolutionary function of dreaming: evidence from dreams of traumatized children. Conscious Cogn 2005;14(1):188–218.

35. Hartmann E, Basile R. Dream imagery becomes more intense after 9/11/01. Dreaming 2003;13(2): 61–6.

36. Hartmann E, Zborowski M, Rosen R, et al. Contextualizing images in dreams: more intense after abuse and trauma. Dreaming 2001;11(3):115–26.

37. Kaminer H, Lavie P. Sleep and dreaming in Holocaust survivors: dramatic decrease in dream recall in well-adjusted survivors. J Nerv Ment Dis 1991; 179(11):664–9.

38. Lavie P, Kaminer H. Sleep, dreaming, and coping style in Holocaust survivors. In: Barrett D, editor. Trauma and dreams. Cambridge (MA): Harvard University Press; 1996. p. 114–24.

39. Lavie P, Kaminer H. Dreams that poison sleep: dreaming in Holocaust survivors. Dreaming 1991; 1(1):11–21.

40. Germain A, Nielsen TA. Sleep pathophysiology in posttraumatic stress disorder and idiopathic nightmare sufferers. Biol Psychiatry 2003;54(10):1092–8.

41. Mellman TA, Hipolito MM. Sleep disturbances in the aftermath of trauma and posttraumatic stress disorder. CNS Spectr 2006;11(8):611–5.

42. Mellman TA, Kulick-Bell R, Ashlock LE, et al. Sleep events among veterans with combat-related posttraumatic stress disorder. Am J Psychiatry 1995; 152(1):110–5.

43. Krakow B, Tandberg D, Barey M, et al. Nightmares and sleep disturbance in sexually assaulted women. Dreaming 1995;5(3):199–206.

44. Pynoos RS, Frederick C, Nader K, et al. Life threat and posttraumatic stress in school-age children. Arch Gen Psychiatry 1987;44(12):1057–63.

45. McCahill TW, Meyer LC, Fischman A. The aftermath of rape. Lexington (MA): Lexington Books; 1979.

46. Terr LC. Chowchilla revisited: the effects of psychic trauma four years after a school-bus kidnapping. Am J Psychiatry 1983;140(12):1543–50.

47. Terr LC. Children of Chowchilla: a study of psychic trauma. Psychoanal Study Child 1979;34:547–623.

48. Coalson B. Nightmare help: treatment of trauma survivors with PTSD. Psychother Theor Res Pract Train 1995;32(3):381–8.

49. Mellman TA, David D, Kulick-Bell R, et al. Sleep disturbance and its relationship to psychiatric morbidity after Hurricane Andrew. Am J Psychiatry 1995;152(11):1659–63.

50. Krakow B, Haynes PL, Warner TD, et al. Clinical sleep disorder profiles in a large sample of trauma survivors: an interdisciplinary view of posttraumatic sleep disturbance. Sleep and Hypnosis 2007;9(1): 6–15.

51. Esposito K, Benitez A, Barza L, et al. Evaluation of dream content in combat-related PTSD. J Trauma Stress 1999;12(4):681–7.

52. Pynoos RS, Nader K. Children who witness the sexual assault of their mothers. J Am Acad Child Adolesc Psychiatry 1988;27(5):567–72.

53. Terr LC. Psychic trauma in children: observations following the Chowchilla school-bus kidnapping. Am J Psychiatry 1981;138(1):14–9.

54. Kravitz M, McCoy BJ, Tompkins DM, et al. Sleep disorders in children after burn injury. J Burn Care Rehabil 1993;14(1):83–90.

55. Eudell EM. Content analysis of dreams following the September 11th terrorist attacks: assessment of interpersonal functioning and stress reactions [unpublished doctoral dissertation]. New York: Adelphi University; 2004.

56. Wilmer HA. The healing nightmare: war dreams of Vietnam veterans. In: Barrett D, editor. Trauma and dreams. Cambridge (MA): Harvard University Press; 1996. p. 85–99.

57. Waiess EA. The traumatic dreams of battered women: a study of after-effects in women who have left battering relationships [unpublished doctoral dissertation]. Central Michigan University; 1997.

58. Horowitz FD. Developmental perspectives on child and adolescent posttraumatic stress disorder. J Sch Psychol 1996;34(2):189–91.

59. Hartmann E. Dreams and nightmares: the new theory on the origin and meaning of dreams. New York: Plenum Trade; 1998.

60. Schreuder BJ, Egmond V, Kleijn WC, et al. Daily reports of post-traumatic nightmares and anxiety dreams in Dutch war victims. J Anxiety Disord 1998;12(6):511–24.

61. van der Kolk B, Blitz R, Burr W, et al. Nightmares and trauma: a comparison of nightmares after combat with lifelong nightmares in veterans. Am J Psychiatry 1984;141(2):187–90.

62. Nader K, Pynoos R, Fairbanks L, et al. Children's PTSD reaction one year after a sniper attack at their school. Am J Psychiatry 1990;147(11): 1526–30.

63. Levine JB. The role of culture in the representation of conflict in dreams: a comparison of Bedouin, Irish, and Israeli children. J Cross Cult Psychol 1991; 22(4):472–90.

64. Punamaki R-L. The role of dreams in protecting psychological well-being in traumatic conditions. Int J Behav Dev 1998;22(3):559–88.

65. Nielsen TA, Stenstrom P. What are the memory sources of dreaming? Nature 2005;437(7063): 1286–9.

66. Hartmann E, Zborowski M, Kunzendorf R. The emotion pictured by a dream: an examination of emotions contextualized in dreams. Sleep and Hypnosis 2001;3(1):33–43.

67. Hartmann E, Brezler T. A systematic change in dreams after 9/11/01. Sleep 2008;31(2):213–8.

68. Bilu Y. The other as a nightmare: the Israeli-Arab encounter as reflected in children's dreams in Israel and the West Bank. Polit Psychol 1989; 10(3):365–89.

69. Garfield P. Nightmares in the sexually abused female teenager. Psychiatr J Univ Ott 1987;12(2):93–7.

70. Fernandez ME. Dreams and nightmares among university women with a history of sexual abuse [unpublished doctoral dissertation]. Carleton University; 1991.

71. Cuddy MA. Predicting sexual abuse from dissociation, somatization and nightmares [unpublished doctoral dissertation]. York University, Toronto, Canada; 1990.

72. Ellenson GS. Detecting a history of incest: a predictive syndrome. Soc Casework 1985;66(4): 525–32.

73. Wright J, Koulak D. Dreams and contemporary stress: a disruption-avoidance-adaptation model. Sleep 1987;10(2):172–9.

74. Arvanitakis K, Jodoin R, Lester E, et al. Early sexual abuse and nightmares in the analysis of adults. Psychoanal Q 1993;62(4):572–87.

75. Fernandez ME, Cuddy MA, Hoffmann RF, et al. Dreams and nightmares among university women with a history of sexual abuse. Paper presented at Annual International Conference of the Association for the Study of Dreams. Charlottesville (VA), June 24–29, 1991.

76. Cuddy M, Belicki K. Predicting a history of sexual abuse from nightmares. Can Psychol 1990;31:384.

77. King J, Sheehan JR. The use of dreams with incest survivors. In: Barrett D, editor. Trauma and dreams. Cambridge (MA): Harvard University Press; 1996. p. 56–67.

78. Pynoos RS, Steinberg AM, Piacentini JC. A developmental psychopathology model of childhood traumatic stress and intersection with anxiety disorders. Biol Psychiatry 1999;46(11):1542–54.

79. Rofe Y, Lewin I. Daydreaming in a war environment. J Ment Imagery 1980;4:59–75.

80. Moffitt A, Kramer M, Hoffmann R. The functions of dreaming. Albany (NY): State University of New York Press; 1993.

81. Diekelmann S, Wilhelm I, Born J. The whats and whens of sleep-dependent memory consolidation. Sleep Med Rev 2009;13(5):309–21.

82. Stickgold R. EMDR: a putative neurobiological mechanism of action. J Clin Psychol 2002;58(1):61–75.

83. Nielsen T, Levin R. Nightmares: a new neurocognitive model. Sleep Med Rev 2007;11(4):295–310.

Dreaming Epiphenomena of Narcolepsy

Lawrence Scrima, PhD, DABSM

KEYWORDS

- Dreaming • Mentation • REM sleep
- REM sleep-related phenomena
- Cataplexy • Narcolepsy

What can dreaming, an epiphenomenon of rapid eye movement (REM) sleep, reveal under normal and abnormal conditions? Is the process of dreaming merely a psychophysiologic process that produces hallucinatory activity, or does the process of dreaming serve adaptive-survival functions? This article examines some of the neuromechanisms associated with dreaming and some of the evidence for the importance of dreaming, by examining a sleep disorder characterized by intense REM sleep and dreaming (ie, narcolepsy). Some evidence for dreaming as a process that may improve adaptive behavior, by integrating memories, motivations, and emotions, is discussed in light of research with narcolepsy patients and their response to a nontraditional treatment. Some experimental methods are described that may be productive for dreaming research, to study it more directly, to derive more information, and to gain more insight into its functions and underlying neuromechanisms.

NARCOLEPSY

The study of sleep has helped elucidate brain neuromechanisms that are actively responsible for the different states of consciousness, wakefulness and sleep, as well as non-REM (NREM) sleep and REM sleep.[1] The study of narcolepsy has focused on understanding and treating the various symptoms of this disorder and thereby continues to advance the understanding of brain mechanisms related to consciousness, alertness, sleep, NREM sleep, REM sleep, and REM sleep-related phenomena as well as neurochemical mechanisms that support these states.[1–6] A clear understanding of how narcolepsy is defined is first necessary.

Narcolepsy is a disorder that presents with several physiologic and psychological characteristics, some of which are relatively well understood and others that are still being studied by researchers from psychology, psychiatry, neurology, and neuroscience. Narcolepsy was described by Gelineau in 1880 as a "neurosis" and consequently was first researched and treated by psychiatrists, as has been recently described.[7] Narcolepsy is currently defined and summarized in the International Classification of Sleep Disorders[8] as a neurologic disorder, primarily characterized by recurring excessive sleepiness, usually relieved by short refreshing naps, and either with or without cataplexy (the sudden loss of muscle tone in response to strong emotion). A diagnosis of narcolepsy, with or without cataplexy, must be objectively confirmed with a positive multiple sleep latency test (MSLT), preceded by a diagnostic overnight polysomnogram, because other sleep disorders share some of its characteristics. The MSLT is a series of daytime nap tests, starting 1.5 to 3 hours after an overnight polysomnogram test, with each nap opportunity lasting 15 to 30 minutes and repeated four to five times, every 2 hours. For a diagnosis of narcolepsy, two or more naps must contain REM sleep and a short latency to sleep onset of 8 minutes or less. Sleep apnea patients often have MSLT results positive for hypersomnolence and sometimes a false-positive for narcolepsy, apparently from REM sleep deprivation, especially in cases where frequent

Sleep-Alertness Disorders Center-Consultants, 1390 South Potomac Street, Suite 110, Aurora, CO 80012, USA
E-mail address: scrimasleepdoc@MSN.com

Sleep Med Clin 5 (2010) 261–275
doi:10.1016/j.jsmc.2010.01.011

apneas occur during REM sleep. In the latter case, this usually remits when sleep apnea is effectively treated, unless narcolepsy is a comorbid disorder.

Besides excessive daytime sleepiness and cataplexy, symptoms of narcolepsy can include one or more of the following: daytime "sleep attacks" with or without REM sleep; other REM sleep phenomena, such as sleep paralysis, hypnagogic hallucinations, and sometimes REM behavior disorder; as well as poor sleep maintenance in about 50% of narcolepsy patients. These REM sleep phenomena can occur in patients without narcolepsy, but they tend to be more frequent and intense in narcoleptics and are viewed as representing REM sleep intrusion into wakefulness. Patients with narcolepsy can also have obstructive sleep apnea, especially if they are overweight, and central sleep apnea comorbidity is also possible, especially with a history of head injury or stroke. There is also some research suggestive of a high comorbidity with periodic limb movement disorder.[9]

Narcolepsy symptoms begin with excessive sleepiness, typically between the ages of 15 and 25 or, in rare cases, even earlier than age 5, and occasionally in senior adults.[8] Usually, cataplexy develops within 5 to 10 years.[10,11] Narcolepsy can be associated with genetic predisposing factors, notably the HLA subtypes DR2/DRB1*1501 and DQB1*0602,[12] but also can be caused by environmental factors. For example, one study of 17 monozygotic twins revealed only 29% of the twins both had narcolepsy-cataplexy, stressing the importance of nongenetic and environmental factors. The most commonly reported medical causes of narcolepsy-cataplexy are head trauma or viral illness, and recently reported streptococcal bacterial infections.[13] Behavioral causes most sited include abrupt change in sleep-wake patterns or sustained sleep deprivation. Other medical and behavioral conditions have also been cited as possible contributors to narcolepsy developing (eg, as reported from a 100-case series).[14]

The impact of narcolepsy on patients untreated or not optimally treated illuminates the importance of normal sleep, including normal REM sleep and dreaming pressure, for healthy physiologic, emotional, and cognitive stability. Narcolepsy patients who are optimally treated describe their life before optimal treatment as having been extremely challenging: coping with continuous or intermittent exhaustion, mental fogginess, feeling "out of it" and socially isolated, unable to sustain reading or concentration, emotionally constrained, and accident-prone. Some characterize it as "feeling like not having slept for 48 hours" or "living in the twilight zone, most of the time."

NARCOLEPSY-CATAPLEXY (DREAMING?) NEUROMECHANISMS
Hypocretin Cell Loss

Among reports suggesting that narcolepsy is associated with a strong pressure for REM sleep and dreaming is one published in 1981 (**Fig. 1**), proposing that narcolepsy is caused by damage to neuromechanisms that suppress NREM sleep and REM sleep during the day.[3] This hypothesis is now supported by research of hypocretin cell loss in narcolepsy patients,[15] as recently reviewed.[2,6] Although the primary neuromechanisms for NREM sleep and REM sleep are different in the brain, they interact[1] in a neurochemical homeostatic way.[6] Because excessive sleepiness is usually the first symptom of narcolepsy and is followed by cataplexy, typically 5 to 10 years later,[10,11] the proposed etiology also hypothesized that the damage to the REM sleep neuromechanism takes longer to occur than the damage to the NREM neuromechanism.[3] In recent years, research has revealed evidence that, for most patients with narcolepsy, the damaged area to the brain associated with promoting hypersomnolence and eventually cataplexy seems to be the area of the posterior hypothalamus that produces hypocretin, also called "orexin," as recently reviewed.[2] These orexin neurons are tonically active during the waking state, decreasing their activity during NREM sleep, and demonstrating the least activity during REM sleep.[2] The evidence suggests that hypocretin cells activate neurons that promote wakefulness and inhibit sleep-activating neurons of the ventrolateral preoptic nucleus.[2] Recent animal research with mice is supportive of the theory that orexin neurons are necessary for circadian control of REM sleep.[16] The die-off of the hypocretin-producing cells is apparently gradual and is probably the most common cause for the progression of hypersomnolence[17] in narcolepsy patients. When the die-off of the hypocretin cells is farther advanced ($\geq$90%), cataplexy is reported to be more likely to occur,[17] as was generally predicted.[3] This gradual die-off of hypocretin cells is probably why cataplexy onset is usually delayed by years from the onset of excessive sleepiness symptoms[10,11] and why the MSLT test is more sensitive to early diagnosis of narcolepsy developing, than by assessing for hypocretin-1 levels in the cerebral spinal fluid. Without sufficient levels of orexin and through the disinhibition of REM-on cells,[2] fast and sudden transitions from waking to sleep, and direct transition to REM sleep and the REM sleep-related epiphenomena are unapposed, including dreaming.

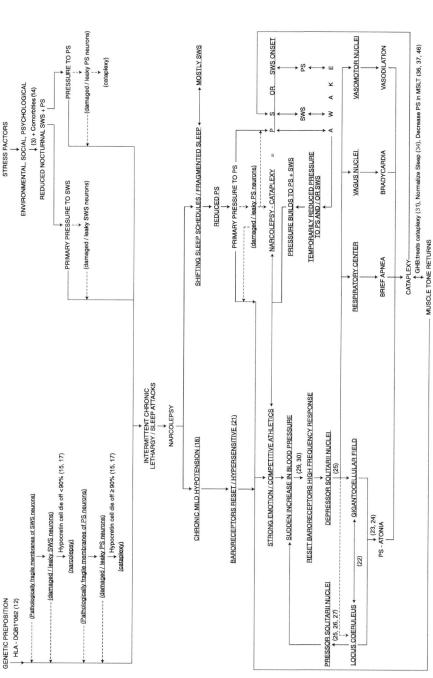

Fig. 1. An Etiology of Narcolepsy-Cataplexy, Updated. The etiology of narcolepsy-cataplexy proposed in 1981 and modified in 1983 with detailed explanations (3, 4), is updated with supporting reports and reference numbers within parentheses. Rapid eye movement (REM) sleep = paradoxical sleep (PS), non-REM (NREM) sleep = slow wave sleep (SWS). Those components that have well demonstrated cause-effect relationships are in capital letters; hypothesized relationships having a causal influence in the development and manifestation of narcolepsy-cataplexy with some supporting evidence are underlined. The solid lines connect components that have some supportive evidence; components within parentheses have tangential or no supporting evidence, are based on plausible conjecture, but are not essential to the proposed etiology. The dashed lines attach conjectural components at plausible junctions. The proposed progression of the cause-effect relationships are indicated by arrows. References from this paper have been added within parentheses (x) on the figure, where applicable.

Factors and neuromechanisms that trigger cataplexy, REM sleep-related phenomena, and dreaming are still being researched. Some of these are described next.

Blood Pressure

That hypersomnolence fosters low blood pressure has been noted off and on since 1934, with this classic literature extensively reviewed in an earlier report.[3] More recently, a retrospective study of 553 narcolepsy patients reported that those who were not obese and were off stimulants, both known to increase blood pressure, had systolic and diastolic blood pressures, respectively, of 0.43 and 0.68 below the standard deviation normative data.[18] A subset of 23 patients of the 553 narcolepsy patients from one site, with only a few overweight subjects, reported to have systolic and diastolic blood pressure means of 1.0 standard deviation below the norms.[19] Similarly, about 23% of upper airway resistance syndrome patients with hypersomnolence have been reported to have hypotension, but not patients with obstructive sleep apnea, also known to promote higher blood pressure.[20] Research on chronic low blood pressure has demonstrated that the baroreceptors reset and become hypersensitive to sudden increase in blood pressure with a larger than normal pressor response.[21] There is evidence from animal studies that the area receiving this pressor response, the solitarii nuclei, have collaterals to other areas of this same nuclei that promote a depressor response to lower blood pressure, which has indirect input by connections to the gigantocellular field,[22] which in turn projects to and receives projections from the locus coeruleus, reported to be involved in propagating the atonia of REM sleep.[23–25] The locus coeruleus has also been reported to elicit a pressor response when stimulated and to modulate the depressor response mechanism in animals; there is some evidence that there are projections of the locus coeruleus that terminate near the solitarii nuclei.[26,27] From these studies, a triggering or contributing neuromechanism of cataplexy in narcolepsy patients was proposed, referred to here as the "pressor trigger of cataplexy" (PTC).[3,4]

The fundamental assumptions and review of the hypothesis and evidence for the PTC are as follows: (1) narcoleptics have a high pressure for REM sleep, promoting a low threshold for REM sleep and REM sleep-related phenomena, including cataplexy; (2) sudden strong emotions cause a sudden strong increase in blood pressure; (3) this stimulates the locus coeruleus, promoting the atonia that occurs during REM sleep and cataplexy; (4) until homeostasis is achieved by blood pressure restabilizing or a reduction of the REM sleep pressure from a nap with REM sleep.

It is well known that cataplexy is triggered by strong emotions and there is evidence that the amygdala is involved in emotional memories, REM sleep, and catapelxy, as recently reviewed.[28] Strong emotions can be assumed to cause a sudden increase in blood pressure.

In 1983, a small pilot study of blood pressure changes during cataplexy was performed,[29] including the beat-to-beat measurements of pulse transit time (PTT). PTT is a highly correlated indirect measure of systolic blood pressure, when averaged over time. PTT measurements were collected and recorded before, during, and after cataplexy events, providing data to test the PTC hypothesis.[3] The four participating narcoleptic patients were off tricyclic antidepressant medications for greater than or equal to 48 hours and off stimulants for greater than or equal to 20 hours, in a repeated measurements design. In addition to PTT, electroencephalogram (EEG), electro-oculogram, chin electromyogram, electrocardiogram, and auto blood pressure (at a rate of one per minute), were recorded and continuously monitored. The patients were monitored and polygraphically recorded for several hours in the afternoon, which included a 10-minute baseline; longer periods of attempts to induce cataplexy (by joking, debating, playing a video game, and so forth); and one or more nap periods. There were only two subjects where blood pressure was captured within the 10 seconds before and during catapelxy events, of which only one had a postcatapelxy measure within 10 seconds. Three of the four subjects had systolic blood pressures well below the normative means and two female subjects were more than 1 standard deviation below the normative means. Most importantly, the PTT mean data provided precataplexy, during cataplexy, and postcataplexy measures, which revealed a significant decrease in PTT (ie, an increase in systolic blood pressure) during greater than or equal to 9 seconds of cataplexy, compared with the baseline before cataplexy (paired t test, $P<.02$). These data[29] support the PTC theory.[3]

Moreover, another study inspired by the PTC theory involved a trial of a blood pressure stabilizing medication, propranolol at high doses, to see if it treats cataplexy. Propranolol was reported to treat cataplexy, although most narcoleptics could not tolerate the side effects from propranolol at the high doses used.[30] Nonetheless, the propranolol study results also can be interpreted as supporting the proposed sudden PTC.[3]

Because narcoleptics have a strong pressure for REM sleep, REM sleep-related phenomena, and dreaming, their dreams tend to be more intense and memorable, often occurring at sleep onset.[3,8,10] High REM sleep pressure is probably caused by one or more of the following: REM sleep deprivation caused by fragmented sleep, medications, or comorbidities (eg, sleep apnea, periodic limb movement disorder, chronic pain, and so forth) or hypocretin cell loss in the posterior hypothalamus (that inhibits sleep during wakefulness). The PTC theory proposed that narcoleptic patients with a high pressure for REM sleep are at a low threshold for REM sleep, making REM sleep-related phenomena and dreaming more likely to occur with the right precipitating behavior (eg, strong emotion, laughing, anger, surprise, competitive sports, and so forth), triggering a sudden increase in blood pressure.[3,4,18,21,29,30] It is noteworthy that tricyclic antidepressants, which strongly suppress REM sleep, can also increase blood pressure and increase muscle tone, thereby effectively treating cataplexy and REM-related phenomena for the short term, but typically becoming less effective over the long term.[2,3,6,31] The serotonin reuptake inhibitors that have a long half-life (eg, fluoxetine, with its metabolite norfluoxetine, can have a half-life of 2–3 weeks or longer in patients with slower metabolisms) and may have fewer side effects and more delayed habituating effects. When antidepressants are withdrawn without tapering, there is an increase or rebound of cataplexy and REM sleep-related phenomena, and usually an increase in intense to nightmarish dreaming, which gradually subside.[3,32]

γ-Hydroxybutyrate Treatment

γ-Hydroxybutyrate (GHB) is a natural metabolite of γ-aminobutyric acid and is normally produced in the human brain.[33] GHB is the only treatment for cataplexy approved by the Food and Drug Administration. More recently, the Food and Drug Administration also approved GHB for treating the symptom of hypersomnolence in narcoleptics. In the first double-blind clinical trial, patients had a significant increase in deep sleep (stages 3 and 4, now collectively called N3; $P<.05$); fewer awakenings ($P<.05$); fewer stage shifts ($P<.01$); and did not suppress REM sleep, during nocturnal sleep,[34] which was subsequently replicated.[35] GHB promotes more normal sleep in narcoleptics, because it does not suppress REM sleep (at lower doses ~1.5–3 g), decreases arousals, and augments deep sleep. Moreover, there were improvements on daytime sleepiness and REM

pressure, documented in the first double-blind clinical trials, using MSLT tests after 29 days of treatment, which revealed significantly fewer naps with REM sleep ($P<.04$) versus placebo.[36] Even more important, the MSLT results further improved and approached normal values after 4 to 14 months of GHB treatment compared with baseline, with longer sleep-onset latency ($P<.05$); increased awake time during naps ($P<.01$); decreased number of REM naps ($P<.01$); and decreased REM sleep minutes ($P<.02$).[37] Most importantly, GHB was documented to effectively treat narcolepsy and cataplexy in a number of double-blind clinical trials,[31,39] and open label or longitudinal trials for up to 1 to 5 years,[40–43] and for up to 14 years at one site.[44]

Abrupt withdrawal of GHB did not cause REM sleep or cataplexy rebound; rather, cataplexy only gradually returned after several weeks.[31,45] Not only did daytime REM sleep pressure decrease with GHB use,[36,37] but also cataplexy, the other REM sleep-related phenomena, and excessive sleepiness greatly improved.[31,35,38–42,44,46]

Why does GHB work to decrease cataplexy and hypersomnolence? GHB does not suppress NREM or REM sleep during the day, unlike hypocretin. GHB seems to work in one or more ways: indirectly, by simply promoting good quality nocturnal sleep[2,31,32,34]; or directly, as a sleep neurotransmitter or neuromodulator[31,34] that makes up for some deficit, because it normalizes sleep and greatly decreases cataplexy frequency, despite severe loss of hypocretin cells in patients with cataplexy; or by decreasing REM pressure and hypersomnolence sufficiently that patients are able to be more active. Increased activity levels typically help to normalize low blood pressure, allowing the baroreceptors to reset to more normal levels and stop their baroreceptors from being hypersensitive to sudden increases in blood pressure during strong emotions. According to the PCT theory, by removing the two prerequisites for cataplexy (strong pressure for REM sleep and hypersensitive baroreceptors) cataplexy does not occur, despite the severe loss of hypercretin cells. Also of interest is a very detailed review on GHB and narcolepsy with a proposed homeostatic theory, which assembles evidence for GHB as facilitating the normal balance between monaminergic and cholinergic neurotransmitters.[6]

Most relevant to this article is that patients followed closely for up to 14 years on GHB (1985–2000)[40,44] reported no longer having frequent intense dreams or intense hypnogogic hallucinations. A few of these patients, who had reported deriving some entertainment from their intense dreams, expressed some disappointment at their loss, but did not want to go off GHB to let their intense dreams return (author's unpublished data).

GHB Treatment Impact

A number of patients who participated the double-blind trial of GHB[31,34] continued into an open-label GHB study, combining with other patients who joined this study to produce a total of 14 years of longitudinal data with GHB.[40,44] Of these patients, 97% (34 of 35 patients) described their GHB treatment results as having "life altering positive impact."[44] For these narcoleptics, GHB was life altering because it allowed them to sleep more normally, restricting REM sleep-related phenomena and dreaming within the state of sleep, instead of intruding as cataplexy, hallucinations, and sleep attacks, and without or with diminished use of stimulant medication. GHB allowed sleep and dreaming to occur at the end of the day, so that they could awaken refreshed, clearheaded, and emotionally balanced. Many of the narcolepsy patients in this longitudinal study stated that the GHB treatment was "liberating," described in the following ways: enabling them to sleep the night through, other than the brief awakening to take their middle of the night dose, without disturbing dreams or hypnagogic hallucinations on lying down and throughout the night; enabling them to stay awake, maintain concentration to study and work, to seek better jobs, to hold a baby, make love, to express full emotional range without fear of cataplexy; to enjoy seeing a movie, play, or other activity all the way to the end without cataplexy or falling asleep; enabling them to be free of humiliating and expensive emergency services (for public cataplexy attacks, often prolonged because of embarrassment); enabling them to have confidence to accomplish tasks without disruptive or dangerous cataplexy or sleep attacks (eg, cooking, studying, reading a book, attending their children's play).

One grade school teacher, who had participated in my narcolepsy memory narcoleptic approach paradigm (NAP) study before she started on GHB, kept a constant tight reign on her emotions to prevent cataplexy while teaching and throughout the day. I recalled her face as very stern, very angular. After being on GHB for several months, she stopped by the sleep laboratory and I did not recognize her until she introduced herself. Her face was transformed: all stern angles rounded out. She described how much she was now enjoying being able to keep up with and laugh with her students. Removal of the fear of cataplexy

had transformed her life, her personality, and even her looks.

For some patients, the mere diagnosis of narcolepsy was life altering, especially those who had been stigmatized by their family and acquaintances for their "invisible problems." Most had been stigmatized as "lazy," "weird," "on drugs," or "crazy," and some recalled their dismay at being told by their doctor that they were "malingering" or having "psychiatric problems." This social stigma had been very disturbing for patients. One young woman, who developed narcolepsy with cataplexy in high school, recalled being accused of taking drugs by her instructor, during a prolonged cataplexy attack in gym class; an ambulance was called and disciplinary procedures against her relating to drug suspicions were initiated. Another young woman, from an evangelical family, was raised to believe that her symptoms were a sign that she was possessed by the devil. For these patients, the narcolepsy diagnosis provided relief from fear of their symptoms, relief from feelings of irrational guilt, and relief from the humiliation of social stigma.

Yet another young woman, a Native American, had inadequately treated narcolepsy that prevented her from normal daily activities, study, work, and participation in tribal ceremonies, because of lack of the necessary physical stamina, cataplexy, and alertness. She had been declared totally disabled (classified as "nonrehabilitatible"). With GHB, she was able to maintain alertness, to study and use a computer, and was able to complete graduate studies. Before GHB treatment, her friends used to hover around her to intervene if she had a cataplexy attack (eg, while cooking, walking, and so forth), whereas on GHB she became fully independent and was able to enjoy normal life activities, including "the joy of full participation in cultural and spiritual ceremonies."

Indeed, many narcolepsy patients who were successfully treated with GHB commented on the fact that they had to develop a new self-image and that friends and family had to develop a new relationship with them, relaxing overprotective habits. Nearly all the GHB longitudinal patients expressed profound appreciation of their new ability to maintain alertness and their freedom from intrusive cataplexy, hypnagogic hallucinations, and intense dreams into their daytime life. Some likened it to emerging from a fog, or to "walking out of darkness into the sunshine." From their experience with renewed normal sleep, one gains more appreciation of the importance of sleep and normal REM sleep and dreaming as a necessary basis for stable emotional, social, and cognitive functioning.

Finally, another memorable narcolepsy patient, seen in 1995, had been on antidepressants for cataplexy for several years. He reported that the antidepressant he was taking had stopped working and that he had developed REM behavior disorder, to the point that his wife would not sleep in the same bed with him. After taking GHB for a few months and also treating his obstructive sleep apnea, his cataplexy and REM behavior disorder both gradually decreased and stopped, except for some very mild and short cataplexy twinges, on rare occasions. His remission from cataplexy and REM behavior disorder continued for several years, but eventually he was lost to follow-up. Another case of REM behavior disorder being successfully treated with GHB was recently reported.[38]

GHB treatment for narcolepsy decreases or eliminates daytime REM sleep-related phenomena and intense dreaming and restores good quality nocturnal sleep. The GHB data can be interpreted to mean that the process of dreaming itself is not inherently impaired, fundamentally different, or abnormal for narcoleptics; only that their dreaming is quantitatively different from normal, in terms of intensity and earlier occurrence.

DREAMING AND REM SLEEP PHENOMENA

Narcolepsy symptoms usually start during young adulthood, with disturbed sleep and impaired alertness maintenance, eventually (typically 5–10 years later)[10,11] progressing to the REM sleep-related phenomena of cataplexy; REM sleep onset at night and during naps; sleep paralysis and hypnagogic (at beginning of sleep) or hypnopompic (at the end of sleep) hallucinations; and more vivid intense dreaming. The symptom progression draws attention to the complex nature of this disorder, involving both physiologic and psychological characteristics, making it a fertile disorder for a wide range of research and interdisciplinary study.

Besides chronic, intermittent, excessive daytime sleepiness, REM sleep-related phenomena are the most defining and differentiating characteristic of narcolepsy. Narcoleptics have a strong pressure for REM sleep, evidenced by a much shorter latency from sleep onset to the first REM sleep period than normals, and a predominance of REM sleep during the first half of nocturnal sleep (normally REM sleep dominates during the last half of nocturnal sleep), and often having REM sleep and dreaming during short naps or sleep attack. Although most sleep apnea patients have excessive daytime sleepiness and some also have a strong pressure for REM sleep,

a short latency to REM sleep, and intense dreaming, these abnormalities usually normalize with effective treatment for sleep apnea (eg, with continuous positive airway pressure treatment), unless a comorbid medical condition or other sleep disorder is present. Sleep paralysis and hypnagogic hallucinations at sleep onset and hypnopompic hallucinations on awaking are related to aspects of REM sleep and dreaming, occurring when awake, and during transitions into or out of sleep. Additionally, cataplexy and sleep paralysis share a defining feature with REM sleep, in that there is the same profound loss of muscle tone as occurs during REM sleep. "Hypnagogic hallucination" is a term used to describe the fleeting perceptions or mentations during the transition to sleep that are not story-like or emotional and that are experienced by most people. In the narcoleptic, however, hypnagogic hallucinations are more like very vivid and intense dreams, sometimes with an abrupt onset, making it difficult for the narcoleptic to distinguish them from reality. Although individuals with narcolepsy experience REM sleep-related phenomena intrusion into the awake state, their dreaming seems to be otherwise the same in all respects as normals, except for increased intensity and earlier onset.

DREAMING RESEARCH: REM VERSUS NREM SLEEP

Problems in presenting an all-inclusive definition of dreams have been reviewed.[47] For the purpose of this article, "mentations" generally refer to any perceptual experience during sleep, whereas "dreams" or "dreaming" refer to story-like, emotional, sometimes bizarre mental theater, with the dreamer as an observer or a participant in the movie-like internal drama. In contrast, "NREM mentations" refers to sleep mentations with any of the following characteristics: logical thinking, not story-like, usually lacking emotional content, simple, fragmented, and fleeting perceptions in any sensory modality (most often reported during the transition to sleep onset or from NREM sleep stages, and sometimes reported as dreams). The one exceptional mentation that consistently has an emotional component is night terrors, occurring during or transitioning from deep stage N3 (stages 3 and 4), which are sometimes erroneously reported as a bad dream or as a nightmare. The emotional component is usually only a single terrifying image and there is no story-like quality or REM sleep. A true nightmare, in comparison, is a negative or frightening intense dream with a story-like quality occurring during REM sleep.

There are some intrinsic problems related to the study of dreams, dreaming, REM sleep phenomena, and REM sleep functions, as described in earlier reports.[47,48] Some of these problems are

1. The occurrence of mentations in all sleep stages
2. The subjective and questionable validity of the dream report
3. The problem of defining dreams (eg, isolated fragmented perceptions, logical thoughts, bizarre story-like and emotion-laden content, and single terrifying image)
4. REM sleep normally occurs after a period of NREM sleep and the longest, most intense episodes of REM sleep usually occur in the last hour or two of sustained routine sleep
5. The problem of delineation of qualitative or quantitative differences between mentations from each sleep stage
6. The possible incorporation or contamination of NREM sleep mentation content into post-REM sleep "dream" reports
7. The possible incorporation or contamination of REM sleep dreams into post-NREM "dream" reports.

NAP, NORMAL AM-PM DREAM REPORT, AND THE MSLT

Various research methods are used to study dreaming and the functions of REM sleep and NREM sleep.[47,48] These methods include collecting dream reports after sleep, isolated REM sleep, or NREM sleep; studying the effects of REM sleep deprivation (by waking up the subject at the start of REM sleep or by the use of medications that suppress REM sleep); various sleep disruption or interruption designs; and first half versus second half of sleep designs. Although such methods have provided useful information, each has significant shortcomings that prevent straightforward interpretations of the data obtained. The source of the confounds ranges from ambiguous differentiation between REM sleep and NREM sleep contribution to obtained results; to inadequate control of diverse stressful effects of sleep deprivation and sleep interruption; to the use of different subjects in the experimental and control groups, where large variability between subjects is likely.

One cardinal problem stems from the fact that appreciable amounts of REM sleep occur after one or more periods of NREM sleep, preventing direct isolation of REM sleep. REM sleep and dreams are usually studied indirectly, by obtaining dream reports after combined NREM and REM sleep occurrence or by depriving REM sleep, to observe and test the effects of deprivation and thereby infer the function of REM sleep from what is deficient when it is not permitted to occur. Such procedures do not control for many variables that most certainly affect the data, which require more conjectural interpretation.

A useful research paradigm for the investigation of psychological (eg, dreaming, mentations, hypnagogic, hypnopompic hallucinations, and night terrors) and physiologic (eg, biochemical, cataplexy, REM behavior disorder, sleep paralysis, and so forth) functions of NREM sleep and REM sleep separately must involve isolating REM sleep for direct study, without promoting stress in the subject and without the use of medications that could also confound clear interpretation of the data. Such a paradigm would enable data to be collected before, during, and after isolated REM sleep or isolated NREM sleep, permitting direct physiologic and psychological study and comparisons of these two sleep phases within the same subject and between subjects. The NAP is just such a research design strategy.[48]

With the cooperation of narcoleptics, the NAP method allows direct testing and decreases the variances and confounds already mentioned, allowing researchers to engage in a wide range of studies, including (1) investigations of the significance of REM sleep and dreams and NREM sleep and mentations as related to emotions and emotional stability, (2) effects of NREM sleep versus REM sleep versus both combined on information processing, vigilance, and other aspects of cognitive and motor performance; and (3) the biochemical, biologic, and homeostatic functions or changes during REM sleep and NREM sleep. Moreover, the NAP can be used to study and compare the effect of REM sleep and dreams versus NREM sleep and mentations on emotional stability, mood, preparedness to learn, ability to solve problems, and so forth. Narcoleptics are intermittently drowsy, can go to sleep very quickly during the day, typically are accustomed to their usual sleep needs, can function for most research purposes without medications, and are normal individuals in other regards. Animals with narcolepsy also could conceivably be used for studies using the NAP method. Detailed description of the NAP method with various research designs can be found in the original report of NAP.[48]

Variations of the NAP can be used for research with other clinical and normal populations, because NREM sleep naps and naps with REM sleep, and dream and mentation reports, can be obtained from most people, although less frequently throughout the day than with narcoleptics.

Most researchers would agree that what people recall as story-like dreams are most likely to be reported after waking up from REM sleep. This is why narcoleptics may provide one of the best sources for the study of dreaming, because they can have dreaming and REM sleep during short naps, and at the beginning of their nighttime sleep. Indeed, NAP was first proposed for the direct study of dreaming and REM sleep functions and used in a study of the effects of isolated REM sleep versus NREM sleep on recall of complex associative information.[48,49]

The NAP approach to research design is able to take advantage of the fact that narcoleptics dream at, or soon after, sleep onset during about 50% of their naps, enabling the researcher to wake the patient up and collect a dream report before other sleep stages occur, except some stage N1 sleep in some naps and stage N2 in even fewer naps. Narcoleptics typically can relate their vivid dreams when they are awakened, whereas most people tend to forget their dreams soon after waking up in the morning. This makes dream recall later in the day from nonnarcoleptics difficult for a researcher directly collecting the dream report and also reviewing them from dream diaries, which are often not written down immediately after waking in the morning. Perhaps narcoleptics remember their dreams better than most people, because they have them soon after sleep onset, but also because their dreams seem to be consistently intense. Moreover, mentations recalled after NREM sleep (including hypnagogic and hypnopompic mentations) also can be studied using NAP design options. The NAP paradigm includes strategies that help to time narcoleptic naps, to predict better the likelihood of naps with or without REM sleep.[48]

A NAP design with normal adult or child subjects is proposed here: the normal AM-PM dream report (NAPDR) design, modeled after the NAP. The NAPDR provides similar advantages to the NAP method over the usual dream collection procedures. The NAPDR schedules early morning naps, to more likely capture REM sleep, and afternoon naps to more likely capture NREM sleep. The wake-up time and the nap duration should be kept fixed for all subjects for each study, with only one nap scheduled per day and dream or mentation reports, performance tests, or recall tests collected immediately on awakening of the subject (or patient fills out a self-report log).

The AM nap could be scheduled for as early in the morning as can be arranged. For example, the subjects could be instructed to set their alarm for 60 minutes earlier than their usual wake-up time (to be somewhat REM sleep deprived); then take a nap at a scheduled time later that morning (may have a performance task to do before the nap); then complete a dream or mentation report immediately on awakening from the nap (may have performance task or test after the nap). Or, they may set an alarm to wake them 1 hour before their usual wake-up time, (may do a performance task), then go back to sleep, and when they wake up again, write down their dream report and do their performance test or recall test. Alternatively, they could wake up at their usual time and take a morning nap at a scheduled time (may have a performance task before the nap) or come straight to the sleep laboratory after getting up (either at usual wake up time or an hour earlier than usual) to do their performance task and have a polysomnogram-recorded nap (to verify sleep and sleep stages during the nap), followed by their dream or mentation report or performance or recall test. These strategies should increase the likelihood of predicting and obtaining REM sleep and dreaming, with subsequent dream reports with minimal NREM sleep on at least some of the sessions in normal subjects. The later in the day a nap is scheduled, the less likely REM sleep occurs.

The PM nap is scheduled for the afternoon, to increase the likelihood of a NREM nap, with the same procedures of mentation or dream report collection afterward and other performance tests as needed. Because AM and PM naps would be scheduled on different days, subjects should be instructed to have the same morning wake-up time for each nap test day, and the duration of the naps should all be the same.

The NAPDR strategy uses a within subject, repeated measures design, to study better the effects of mentation and dream content, relevance, and differences between NREM sleep mentations reports and REM sleep dream reports, or performance tests, evaluating both within and between subjects data. Moreover, the NAPDR design enables assessment of factors that may allow better prediction of the likelihood of NREM sleep and REM sleep (eg, the duration since the last sleep, time of day the nap occurs, amount of emotional or physical stress that occurred preceding the nap, and so forth). These factors helped in predicting the relative likelihood of obtaining a nap with REM sleep or NREM sleep in narcoleptics, as described in the NAP paper,[48] and likely can be useful in the same way for normal subjects using NAPDR.

The MSLT, used to assess objectively the severity of hypersomnolence and assess or rule out narcolepsy developing, even before cataplexy manifestation, can be another method of collecting dream reports,[50] and used to evaluate differences between hypersomnolent types. The frequency of dreaming may have diagnostic screening use for narcolepsy among hypersomnolent patients. One study recently reported that among a sample of 28 hypersomnolent patients reporting dream recall of greater than or equal to one per week, 13 of these patients or 46.4% were noted to meet criteria for narcolepsy with at least two sleep-onset REM periods. In contrast, in the sample of 13 hypersomnolent patients reporting dream recall at less than or equal to one per month, only two of these patients or 15.4%, were found to meet criteria for narcolepsy. If this research is reliably replicated with larger samples, dream recall frequency of greater than or equal to one per week may have a screening potential for narcolepsy developing among hypersomnolent patients, whereas hypersomnolent patients reporting low dream recall ($\leq$one per month) seem to be much less likely to meet criteria for the diagnosis of narcolepsy.[51]

NAP TEST OF REM SLEEP AND DREAMING ON MEMORY

The experience and characteristics of dreaming in narcoleptics seems to be the same as in other people, except that their dreaming tends to be more intense and occur earlier in sleep. In light of the problems of investigating the effects of sleep on learning and memory, especially NREM versus REM sleep, a dissertation was done using a NAP strategy for a sleep memory study.[48,49,52] The research was inspired by the neuronal activity correlates (NAC) theory of information processing,[49] which is based on the premise that neuronal activity (EEG) of wakefulness is correlated with information processing (ie, low-voltage fast-mixed frequency EEG activity). REM sleep EEG, being more like awake EEG, is more likely to support complex information processing and mentations, associated with low-amplitude, mixed-frequency EEG waves, with some theta and alpha waves, whereas NREM sleep, having high-amplitude, slower delta EEG waves (N3) or spindle EEG waves, being less like awake EEG, is more likely to be associated with noncomplex mentations. The NAC theory was proposed to predict differential effects of wakefulness, REM sleep, and NREM sleep on memory. Based on these associations and some of the past research findings, the dissertation proposed to study directly the effect of REM sleep on information processing. It was hypothesized that (1) recall of a complex associative memory task should be best after naps that contain REM sleep; (2) NREM sleep should passively facilitate memory, by preventing retroactive interference; and (3) wakefulness should be the most likely to promote retroactive interference and should produce the lowest memory performance, compared with REM sleep or NREM sleep.[49]

Ten narcoleptics participated in the 16-session study, which took place on 16 different days (24 or more hours apart), with each learning task taking about 10 minutes. One task was a complex associative memory task, solving anagrams (of which there were eight different sets). The other task was a rote learning memory task called trigrams (all consonant capital letters [eg, CZT]), of which there were eight different sets. The anagrams task was the complex associative memory task, consisting of 10 sets of five-letter anagrams with only two possible word solutions (eg, anagram "edcta" solutions: acted, cadet). One set of 10 anagrams was presented per session, with 1-minute exposure to each anagram. When the narcoleptic found a word in the anagram, they were instructed to say the word out loud, spell it, and think of the word in some personal context before continuing with the task and search for the second word, until the minute exposure was finished and then proceed to the next anagram, while the investigator recorded the solutions. The trigram task was the rote memory task, consisting of eight different sets of eight trigrams. The task was presented in a deck of self-paced serial learning, where the subject would try to anticipate the subsequent trigram by spelling it out loud while looking at a blank card on top of each trigram, before looking at the card with the trigram. The deck was recycled until the patient had memorized all the trigrams in order. The trigram task produced a ceiling in recall across all three conditions, and was deemed to be not difficult enough.

The narcoleptics were prepared for polysomnogram monitoring to detect sleep onset and sleep stages, before exposure to the memory task; then, they either took a nap for 20 minutes or remained awake playing the card game "war" with the investigator for 20 minutes without talking and were instructed to avoid rehearsing their found anagram words or trigrams during the game. During the nap condition, their sleep was polygraphically recorded; then, they were awakened and told only to think of the task solutions. After 3 minutes of waking-up time, the subject was then asked to say and spell the anagram solution words (or trigrams) that they recalled. They were given 6 minutes of free recall test time. Sometimes they would recount a dream that would involve the words from the anagram task and, on rare occasion, would recount a new solution to an anagram that they had not found during their original exposure. One patient was under a lot of stress and had nightmares during almost every REM nap; but the data were nonetheless included in the analysis. After the awake session, the subjects were given the same instructions before obtaining their free recall test.

Free recall of the anagram solutions was significantly different between the three different states of consciousness (awake, NREM sleep, and REM sleep), but free recall of the trigram task was not different between the three states of consciousness. For the anagram task, a significant linear relationship was also found ($P<.05$), where recall of anagram solutions after the awake session had the lowest mean (26.1%), after NREM naps the second lowest mean (46.2%), and after naps with REM sleep the highest mean (69.1%) of the anagram solutions.[49] Moreover, there were significant differences between these three states of consciousness. Recall of the anagram solutions after a nap with REM was significantly better than after either a nap with only NREM ($P<.05$) or the awake condition ($P<.01$); NREM recall was significantly better than the awake condition ($P<.05$); and recall of the combined NREM and REM sessions was significantly better than the awake ($P<.01$), for the controlled intersleep interval data.[49]

This study was the first direct human evidence to support the theory that REM sleep (and by association dreaming) is important and probably actively involved in memory of complex associative information, perhaps by some integrating process. The data were interpreted as also supporting the passive theory of why sleep, especially NREM sleep, versus an equal period of wakefulness, repeatedly has been found to improve recall of information, possibly by preventing retroactive interference, the usual explanation of why sustained wakefulness produces the lowest scores on recall tests.[49,52]

Two recent similar findings, using a nap method with normal subjects, found that REM sleep improves creativity by priming associative networks[53] and by consolidating emotional human memories with implications for affective disorders.[54] Overall, these data collectively offer compelling support for the NAC theory, as applied to complex associative information.

ALTERNATIVE THEORIES OF DREAMING

Some have emphasized the visual hallucinatory and delusional quality of dreams.[55] If dreaming is basically a perceptual hallucination, propagated by the ponto-geniculate-occipital neuronal spike-like volleys, which occur during REM sleep and exciting neuronal activity randomly to produce the delusional and hallucinatory experience, then dreaming can be considered as a meaningless, perceptual state.[55] This theory of dreaming does not explain, however, why dreams are so often about our current concerns, nor why early night dreams are mostly about current concerns, middle of the night dreams about older experiences and concerns, and just before waking dreams are again predominately about current concerns.[56] The temporal pattern does not seem to be a random stimulation, nor one attributable to intensity, assuming that higher-intensity dreams trigger older memories, because the most intense dreams tend to occur just before waking, which are typically about current concerns. If the hallucination theory of dreaming were correct, dreams should always be a random sampling of memories, triggered by ponto-geniculate-occipital activity and not consistently show a temporal, story-like, and cogent emotional pattern, nor developmental differences in dreams, problem solving, or helping to resolve emotional issues.

The hallucination theory of dreaming has been used by others to support a theory of dreams as a process of erasure of memories,[57] rather than a source of creative information processing and memory consolidation. Taken to its logical conclusion, the erasure theory would predict that the more we dream, the less we would retain in memory. Further, its presumption that "unimportant" things are erased, belies the fact that we learn a great deal through schooling or general experience that seems unimportant at the time, but later acquires importance through new experience, new motivations, or additional knowledge, when we may experience an "aha" moment as we appreciate the new value of previously "unimportant" or "not interesting" information in our memory that was otherwise "forgotten."

The available evidence instead supports dreaming as a mechanism of experiential integration, memory consolidation, and creative processing. The neurosurgeon Wilder Penfield reported in 1954 that when mildly stimulating different areas of the brain to locate epilepsy-inducing areas that needed to be removed to prevent disabling seizures, he found that certain brain sites elicited very detailed old vivid memories, sometimes "forgotten" vivid memories, being reported as though the patients were reliving detailed minutes of their past experience.[58] This supports the idea that he championed, that even old memories, without apparent importance, may be in long-term storage, without erasure, for decades. Penfield[58] proposed that the brain may record everything it perceives, for the healthy life of the brain. Although critics have claimed that such re-called memories could be just fantasies or halluci-nations, this criticism is countered by the fact that the same memory is re-elicited when the same site is stimulated, that some of the memories were substantiated, and that many have experienced sudden recall of experiences from the remote past at one time or another.

IMPLICATIONS AND NEW METHODS

From sleep and dreaming research, the following implications have some support. (1) Dreaming may have an integrative function for experiences and concerns, possibly prioritizing them, based on emotional importance, through a kind of divergent thinking, to strive for creative solutions to current concerns and problems, to optimize adaptive behavior. (2) Dreaming may provide a mechanism of integration, personifying or "weaving-in" of new experiences with older experiences,[59] to allow cohesive expansion of growing neural networks or tapestry of experience that is the mind. (3) Dreams may provide a way of refreshing old memories, while integrating them with new ones for personi-fying, creative, emotional, and adaptive needs.

The research findings concerning dreaming, dream content, and its apparent importance to the central nervous system, adaptive behavior, emotional stability, and progressive cognitive growth have increasingly elevated its importance in the last several decades. Moreover, the NAC theory and the evidence of the importance of REM sleep and dreaming support a goal of devel-oping medications that do not suppress REM sleep, especially for treatment of medical disor-ders that require chronic use of such medications. Objective assessment of drugs altering normal sleep effects in clinical trials of all medications that affect the central nervous system and sleep function may be prudent. The new treatment GHB with its normalizing effect on the nocturnal sleep of narcolepsy patients, treating cataplexy and decreasing dreaming intensity, despite the profound loss of hypocretin cells, has raised the bar for promoting good quality sleep over the long term.

There are new methods for studying the brain with potential for studying narcolepsy and dreaming, with some new discoveries. Because strong emotions precipitate cataplexy and the emotional link to dreaming, the limbic system, particularly the amygdala (associated with emotional memories), and hippocampus (associ-ated with locating long-term memories), there is interest in studying multiple regions of the brain and how they interact. Magnetic resonance spectroscopy and neuroimaging techniques[60] and other combined behavioral and neurophysio-logical methods may help to further define the role of memory and brain plasticity to elucidate this process.[61] A recent report[62] detailed a study of the integrity of the amygdala and the hypothal-amus and pontomesencephalic junction in narco-lepsy patients using magnetic resonance spectroscopy examining the single region, creating an energy spectrum where the peaks correspond to the unique resonance frequency of each chemical in that region, with the following discoveries: decrease in myoinositol in the right amygdala of narcolepsy patients compared with controls was reported; increased activity in the nucleus accumbens, which is a destination for neurons in the mesolimbic dopaminergic pathway, was also reported; dopamine levels in the nucleus accumbens decreased during NREM sleep and re-turned to waking levels during REM sleep, concluding that this area may also be involved in narcolepsy. "While emotions do not trigger REM sleep per se, dreams do trigger emotions, and perhaps the associated limbic structures trigger the muscle atonia of REM sleep. If emotions affect the same motor neurons that are involved in cata-plexy, then perhaps this is why emotions trigger cataplexy."[62]

Tangentially, it has been reported that the effect of bilateral lesioning of the basolateral amygdala in rats impaired ability to demonstrate preference for the high reward versus a low reward alley by faster running time compared with sham lesioned rats.[63] The amygdalectomized rats performed equally bad in both reward alleys, while being partially food deprived. But even more striking was that the amygdalectomized rats did not seem to learn nor care that either alley had food at the end of it, often stopping part way down the alley, looking around, then sauntering on. Without the basolater-al amygdala, motivation seemed to be lost; there was either no motivation to learn or there was impairment in ability to apply past knowledge to obtain the needed goal or both.

Perhaps dreaming serves as a conduit between biologic drives and emotional memories, current motivations and cognitive functions, attempting to resolve emotional issues, problems, and ambigui-ties in life through dreaming. If dreaming serves to integrate, increase associations, and personify all our experiences, to prepare us better for goal-directed behaviors, problems solving, and adaptive behavior, the importance of dreaming should be greatly elevated. What if REM sleep deprivation blocks input of emotional memories from the amyg-dala, so that we lose touch with our purpose in life as individuals? If someone is sleep or REM sleep deprived and these proposed functions of dreaming and REM sleep are at least partly correct, then there would likely be symptoms of automatic behavior, aimless or careless or "care less" behavior or decreased motivation. These kinds of behaviors certainly are often used to describe sleep-deprived people, hypersomnolent patients (eg, sleep apnea patients); and narcoleptics.

REM sleep deprivation may not be the best long-term treatment approach for chronic problems, in light of the accumulating research supporting the importance of REM sleep and dreaming for normal physiologic and psychological functioning, including memory and adaptive behavior. It has been reported that short-term REM sleep deprivation of depressed patients decreases their depression.[64] Such research findings are supportive of the development of antidepressant medications that are strongly REM sleep suppressing. Among the reported side effects of antidepressants, however, are increased risk of developing neurologic tics or tardive dyskinesia, loss of libido, insomnia, hypersomnolence, impotency, suicide, and violent impulses.[65] It is interesting to note that the sleep normalizing biochemical GHB has been reported to treat depression[6] and narcolepsy,[6,31,41] without suppressing REM sleep in the lower dose range (1.5–3.0g).[34]

SUMMARY

Dreaming as epiphenomena of narcolepsy has inspired much diverse research, from medical to behavioral to neuroscience. Dreaming has been the main clue revealing sleep as a mentally active time, when catharsis, inspiration, and memories may be integrated to optimize adaptive behavior, in addition to the quiescent time of nondream or NREM sleep that our bodies need for primarily physiologic renewal. When dreaming is suppressed for long periods by stress, too little sleep, sleep apnea, medications, or hypocretin cell loss, then dream intensity increases; latency from sleep onset to the first REM sleep episode of the night decreases (as in narcolepsy, depression, and sleep apnea); and other REM sleep-related phenomena increase, including hypnagogic and hypnopompic hallucinations, sleep paralysis, and REM behavior disorder. When greater than 90% of the hypocretin cells are lost, cataplexy usually starts to occur.[17] There may be physiologic importance for REM sleep for neurochemical homeostasis (eg, balance between monaminergic and cholinergic neurotransmission).[6] REM sleep may be important for maintaining optimal levels of certain neurochemicals (eg, γ-aminobutyric acid, aspartic acid, and

acetylcholine levels in the frontal cortex; γ-aminobutyric acid and aspartic acid in the thalamus and reticular formation), as derived from REM sleep deprivation studies in animals.[66] Newer physiologic techniques[62,67] should be very helpful in elucidating more neurochemical functions of REM sleep and NREM sleep in the future and possible neurochemical correlates to dreaming.

Sleep and memory research indicates that dreaming and REM sleep seem to reflect an ongoing active process that integrates information from our recent and more remote experiences, especially with regard to our current concerns.[56] The dreaming process may enable us to have an ever increasing facility to retrieve memories for adaptive needs, and allow us to have an ever increasing appreciation and comprehension of our seemingly infinitely complex environment and human condition, as higher levels of integration are achieved. Dreaming seems to be important for information processing, divergent thinking, learning, and memory,[49,53,54] with implications for personifying our experiences, psychological stability, adaptive behavior, and survival. That this process is universal among humans, occurs in its greatest quantity and proportion of sleep during infancy and early childhood,[68] and is predominantly an unconscious process is striking testimony to its fundamental importance.

Dreaming, dreams, and REM sleep function can be studied most efficiently and directly with narcoleptic patients within the NAP method, in hypersomnolent patients using the MSLT or NAP, and with normal subjects with the NAPDR. These methods may help increase the understanding of dreams, dreaming, mentations, and the neuromechanisms involved, and with new physiologic techniques, such as quantitative EEG,[67] magnetic resonance spectroscopy, and neuroimaging.[60] Such research may help to find new treatments or preventative approaches for some sleep disorders, psychological disorders, and some learning disorders, and ways to derive the most benefit from our sleep and dreams.

REFERENCES

1. Siegel JM. Brainstem mechanisms generating REM sleep. In: Kryger MH, Roth T, Dement WC, editors. Principles and practice sleep medicine. 3rd edition. Philadelphia: W.B. Saunders Co; 2000. p. 112–54.
2. Didato G, Boili L. Treatment of narcolepsy. Expert Rev Neurother 2009;9(6):897–910.
3. Scrima L. An etiology of narcolepsy—cataplexy and a proposed cataplexy neuromechanism. Int J Neurosci 1981;15:69–86.

4. Scrima L. A proposed etiology and neuromechanism of cataplexy. Sleep 1983;12:282.

5. Mamelak M. A model for narcolepsy. Can J Psychol 1991;45(2):194–220.

6. Mamelak M. Narcolepsy and depression and the neurobiology of gammahydroxybutyrate. Prog Neurobiol 2009;89(2):193–219.

7. Pagel JF, Scrima L. Psychoanalysis and narcolepsy. In: Goswami M, Pandi-Perumal, Thorpy M, editors. Narcolepsy. New York: Springer; 2010. p. 129–34.

8. American Academy of Sleep Medicine. International classification of sleep disorders. In: Sateia MJ, editor. Diagnostic and coding manual. 2nd edition. Westchester (IL): American Academy of sleep Medicine; 2005. p. 79–115.

9. Hartman P, Scrima L. Muscle activity in the legs (MAL) associated with frequent arousals in narcoleptics and OSA patients. Clin Electroencephalogr 1986;17:181–6.

10. Guilleminault C. Cataplexy. In: Guilleminault C, Dement WC, Passouant P, editors. Narcolepsy. New York: Spectrum Publications; 1976. p. 125–44.

11. Scrima L. Lag time between onset of excessive sleepiness and catapelxy in narcolepsy patients. Sleep Res 1991;20:328.

12. Mignot E, Hayduk R, Black J, et al. HLA DQBQ*602 is associated with cataplexy in 509 narcoleptic patients. Sleep 1997;20:1012–20.

13. Aran A, Ling L, Nevsimalova S, et al. Elevated antistreptococcal antibodies in patients with recent narcolepsy onset. Sleep 2009;32(8):979–83.

14. Scrima L, Miller BR. Pre-onset medical and sleep history of 100 narcoleptics. Sleep 1999;22(Suppl):S155.

15. Peyron C, Faraco J, Rogers W, et al. A mutation in early narcolepsy and a generalized absence of hypocretin peptides in human narcolepsy brains. Nat Med 2000;6:991–7.

16. Kantor S, Mochizuki T, Janisiewicz AM, et al. Orexin neurons are necessary for circadian control of REM sleep. Sleep 2009;32(9):1127–34.

17. Thannickal TC, Nienhuis R, Siegel JM. Localized loss of hypocretin (orexin) cells in narcolepsy without cataplexy. Sleep 2009;32(8):993–8.

18. Scrima L, Garlick I, Victor Y, et al. Narcolepsy patients' blood pressure in higher and lower weight groups. Sleep 1998;21(Suppl):53.

19. Scrima L, Garlick I, Victor Y, et al. Narcolepsy patients' blood pressure and pulse. Sleep Res 1996;25:366.

20. Guilleminault C, Faul JL, Stoohs R. Sleep-disordered breathing and hypotension. Am J Respir Crit Care Med 2001;164(7):1242–7.

21. Pickering T, Sleight P. Baroreceptors and hypertension. In: DeJong W, Provoost A, Shapiro A, editors. Progress in brain research: hypertension and brain mechanisms, vol. 47. Amsterdam: Elsevier/North-Holland and Biomedical Press; 1977. p. 43–60.

22. Amatruda T, Black D, McLenna T, et al. Sleep cycle control and cholinergic mechanisms: differential effects of carbachol injections at pontine brain stem sites. Brain Res 1975;98:501–15.

23. Jouvet M. The role of monoamines and acetylcholine containing neurons in the regulation of the sleep waking cycle. Ergebnisse Physiol 1972;64:166–307.

24. Jones B, Harper S, Halaris A. Effects of locus coeruleus lesions upon cerebral monoamine content, sleep-wakefulness states and the response to amphetamine in the cat. Brain Res 1977;124:473–96.

25. Palkovits M, Zaborszky L. Neuroanatomy of central cardiovascular control. Nucleus tractus solitarii: afferent and efferent neuronal connections in relation to the baroreceptor reflex arc. In: DeJong W, Provoost A, Shapiro A, editors. Progress in brain research: hypertension and brain mechanisms, vol. 47. Amsterdam: Elsevier/North-Holland and Biomedical Press; 1977. p. 9–34.

26. Ward D, Gunn C. Locus coeruleus complex: elicitation of the pressor response and a brain stem region necessary for its occurrence. Brain Res 1976;107:401–6.

27. Ward D, Gunn C. Locus coeruleus complex: differential modulation of depressor mechanisms. Brain Res 1976;107:407–11.

28. Schwartz S, Ponz R, Poryazova R, et al. Abnormal activity in hypothalamus and amygdala during humour processing in human narcolepsy with cataplexy. Brain Advance Access published Dec 19, 2007:1–9. DOI:10.1093/brain/awrn292.

29. Scrima L, Hartman P, Anderson J, et al. The relationship of blood pressure and pulse transit time to narcolepsy and cataplexy. Sleep Res 1983;12:283.

30. Meier-Ewert K, Matsubayashi K, Benter L. Propranolol: long-term treatment in narcolepsy-cataplex. Sleep 1985;8:95–104.

31. Scrima L, Hartman P, Johnson FH, et al. Efficacy of gamma—hydroxybutyrate (GHB) vs placebo in treating narcolepsy—cataplexy: double—blind subjective measures. Biol Psychiatry 1989;26:331–43.

32. Thorpy MJ, Goswami, M. Treatment of narcolepsy. In: Thorpy MJ, editor. Handbook of sleep disorders. New York: Informa Health Care; 1990. p. 235–58.

33. Muyard JP, Laborit HM. Gamma-hydroxybutyrate. In: Forrest IS, Usdin E, editors. Psychopharmacology series, volume 2: psychotherapeutic drugs. Part II. Applications. New York: Marcel Dekker; 1977. p. 1339–75.

34. Scrima L, Hartman P, Johnson FH, et al. The effects of gamma—hydroxybutyrate on the sleep of narcolepsy patients: a double—blind study. Sleep 1990;13(6):479–90.

35. Mamelak M, Black J, Montplaisir J, et al. A pilot study on the effects of sodium oxybate on sleep

architecture and daytime alertness in narcolepsy. Sleep 2004;27(7):1327–34.

36. Scrima L, Johnson FH, Thomas EE, et al. Effect of gamma—hydroxybutyrate (GHB) on multiple sleep latency test (MSLT) in narcolepsy patients: a double—blind study. Sleep Res 1990;19:287.

37. Scrima L, Johnson FH, Thomas EE, et al. Effects of gamma—hydroxybutyrate (GHB) on multiple sleep latency test (MSLT) in narcolepsy patients: a long term study. Sleep Res 1990;19:288.

38. Shneerson JM. Case report: successful treatment of REM sleep behavior disorder with sodium oxybate. Clin Neuropharmacol 2009;32(3):158.

39. U.S. Xyrem Multicenter Study Group. A randomized, double-blind, multicenter trial comparing the effects of three doses of orally administered sodium oxybate with placebo for the treatment of narcolepsy. Sleep 2002;25(1):42–9.

40. Scrima L. Gamma-hydroxybutyrate (GHB) treated narcolepsy patients continue to report cataplexy controlled for up to five (5) years. Sleep Res 1992;21:262.

41. U.S. Xyrem Multicenter Study Group. A 12 month, open-label, multicenter extension trial of orally administered sodium oxybate for the treatment of narcolepsy. Sleep 2003;26(1):31–5.

42. U.S. Xyrem Multicenter Study Group. Sodium oxybate demonstrates long-term efficacy for the treatment of cataplexy in patients with narcolepsy. Sleep Med 2004;5:119–23.

43. Broughton R, Mamelak M. The treatment of narcolepsy-cataplexy with nocturnal gamma-hydroxybutyrate. Can J Neurol Sci 1979;6:1–6.

44. Scrima L, Skakich-Scrima S, Miller BR. The efficacy of gamma-hydroxybutyrate (GHB) in narcoleptics: 9 years [abstract]. Sleep 2000;23(Suppl):293.

45. U.S. Xyrem Multicenter Study Group. The abrupt cessation of therapeutically administered sodium oxybate (GHB) does not cause withdrawal symptoms. Clin Toxicol 2003;41:131–5.

46. Scrima L, Shander D. Letter to editor on article: narcolepsy review (Aldrich MS: 8–9–91). N Engl J Med, Medicine 1–24–1991;324(4):270–1.

47. Pagel JF, Blagrove M, Levin R, et al. Definitions of dream: a paradigm for comparing field descriptive specific studies of dream. Dreaming 2001;11(4):194–202.

48. Scrima L. The narcoleptic approach paradigm (NAP) for the direct study of dreams and dream sleep functions. Int J Neurosci 1982;16:69–73.

49. Scrima L. Isolated REM sleep facilitates recall of complex associative information. Psychophysiology 1982;19:252–9.

50. Pagel JF. Sleep stage associated changes in dream recall across the day on awakening from MSLT naps. Sleep 2008;31:A373.

51. Pagel JF, Shocknasse S. Reported dream recall frequency: a marker for sleep onset REMS periods (SORP's) in hypersomnolent patients without OSA [abstract]. Sleep 2007;30(Suppl):214.

52. Scrima L. Dream sleep and memory: new findings with diverse implications. Integr Psychiatry 1984;2:201–40.

53. Cai D, Mednick SA, Harrison EM, et al. REM, not incubation, improves creativity by priming associative networks. Proceedings National Academy of Sciences (PNAS) Early Edition June 8, 2009. Available at: http://www.pnas.org/cgi/10.1073/pnas.0900271106. Accessed May 4, 2009.

54. Nishida M, Pearsall J, Buckner RL, et al. REM sleep, prefrontal theta and the consolidation of human emotional memory. Cereb Cortex 2009;19(5):1158–66.

55. Hobson JA. Abnormal states of consciousness AIM as a diagnostic tool. In Consciousness, vol. 67. New York: Scientific American Library; 1999. p. 188–215.

56. Verdone P. Temporal reference of manifest dream content. Percept Mot Skills 1965;20:1253–68.

57. Crick F, Mitchinson G. The function of dream sleep. Nature 1983;304:111–4.

58. Penfield W. The permanent record of the stream of consciousness. Proceedings of the Fourteenth International Congress of Psychology. Montreal (Canada), June 7–12, 1954. p. 47–69.

59. Hartmann E. Dreaming. In: Lee-Chiong T, Sateia MJ, Carskadon MA, editors. Sleep medicine. Philadelphia: Hanley & Belfus; 2002. p. 93–8.

60. Picchioni D. Commentary on Poryazova R. Using magnetic resonance spectroscopy in narcolepsy to study the limbic mechanisms of cataplexy. Sleep 2009;32(5):581–2.

61. Frank MG, Benington JH. Role of sleep in memory consolidation and brain plasticity: dream or reality? Neuroscientist 2006;12:477.

62. Poryazova R, Schnepf B, Werth E, et al. Evidence for metabolic hypotharmao-amygdala dysfunction in narcolepsy. Sleep 2009;32(5):607–13.

63. Scrima L, Gaston M. Effect of amygdaloid lessons on a differential reward discrimination task [abstracts]. Western Psychological Association. San Francisco (CA): 1974;54:26.

64. Vogel GW, Vogel F, McAbee RS, et al. Improvement of depression by REM sleep deprivation. Arch Gen Psychiatry 1980;37:247–53.

65. Glenmullen J. Prozac backlash. New York: Simon & Schuster; 2000.

66. Freemon R. Sleep research a critical review. Springfield (IL): Charles C. Thomas; 1974. p. 78–81.

67. Kropotov JD. Quantitative EEG event-related potentials and neurotherapy. New York: Elsevier; 2009.

68. Roffwarg H, Muzio J, Dement WC. Ontogenic development of the human sleep-dream cycle. Science 1966;152:604–19.

Drugs, Dreams, and Nightmares

J.F. Pagel, MS, MD[a,b,c],*

KEYWORDS

• Dream • Nightmares • Medications • Parasomnias • PTSD

Medications affect sleep in at least three general ways: (1) altering cognitive levels of sleepiness/alertness, (2) altering cognitive activity during sleep—generally reported as dreaming, or (3) affecting the symptoms of sleep, medical and psychiatric diagnoses known to alter sleep. Although this article addresses how medications affect dreaming and nightmares, the effects that medications have on cognitive activity in sleep are closely associated with medication effects on sleepiness/alertness and on associated diagnoses known to alter sleep.

Until recently, neurochemists interested in dreaming focused their studies on the effects of various neurochemicals on rapid eye movement (REM) sleep based on the belief that medications affecting dreaming would be the same ones known to affect REM sleep. Agents that suppress REM sleep, such as ethanol, and benzodiazepines, such as valium, induce episodes of REM sleep rebound on withdrawal. These REM sleep rebound episodes have been associated with reports of nightmares and disturbed dreaming and were considered the primary mechanism resulting in drug-induced disordered dreaming and nightmares. This approach to studying REM sleep as dreaming had significant research advantages because the specific neurochemical effects of phamachologic agents on REM sleep could be studied in animal models with no dream report required. Over the past 50 years, this theoretic definition of dreaming as REM sleep became the routine approach used in studying dreaming in animal and human central nervous system (CNS) scanning studies. There is little question, however, that dreaming occurs without REM sleep and that REM sleep occurs without reported dreaming.[1–3] There is only limited evidence for any special association between REM sleep and dreaming.[3,4]

Recent studies have looked at the affects of medications on dreaming in human beings, the only species that can currently report the content and an experience of whether or not a dream has occurred. Clinical trials required for the use and release of new agents provide an extensive base of such drug effects and side-effect information. Most such studies are large, specific, and well designed. Physicians in medical practice can also submit case reports of drug side effects for drugs in clinical use. These case reports often address the psychoactive side of particular agents. This information is less specific than that derived from animal studies; however, it has the advantages of large group study size, it is human based, and not limited to known or theoretic effects of particular types of medication. Limitations of this approach include its reliance on human subject reports, limitations in the studies of older agents that are sometimes used in the assessment and approval of current drugs, the lack of such assessments in some clinical trials of agents presumed not to have cognitive side effects, and the fact that such studies are not done on agents not approved for clinical use in the practice of medicine.[5,6] Current knowledge of the psychoactive effects of medications is based on a coupling of this clinical knowledge with specific neurochemical effects that can be studied in animal models.

The pharmachodynamics of psychoactive medications are affected by the half-life of activity, which varies based on gastrointestinal uptake, competition with other agents, and efficacy of

a Department of Family Medicine, School of Medicine, University of Colorado, CO, USA
b Sleep Disorders Center of Southern Colorado, 1619 North Greenwood, Suite 107, CO 81003, USA
c Sleepworks Sleep Laboratory, Colorado Springs, 1330 Quail Lake Loop, CO 80906, USA
* Department of Family Medicine, School of Medicine, University of Colorado, CO, USA.
E-mail address: Pueo34@earthlink.net

Sleep Med Clin 5 (2010) 277–287
doi:10.1016/j.jsmc.2010.01.007
1556-407X/10/$ – see front matter © 2010 Elsevier Inc. All rights reserved.

hepatic or urinary elimination systems. The ability of an agent to cross the blood-brain barrier into the CNS affects the ability of that agent to induce CNS effects and side effects. Once these variables have been addressed, the potential CNS effects of any agent remain complex. It is the rare drug that is a pure agonist for a single neuron type, with most, if not all, medications affecting the binding of multiple CNS neuroreceptors. Neuroreceptors vary locally in concentration and response throughout the CNS. Subtypes exist for each neuroreceptor that vary genetically between individuals as well as locally depending on CNS location. Neurons are likely to respond to multiple neurotransmitters.[7,8] Despite these limitations and the complexity of the applicable neuropharmacology, the primary neuroreceptor effects for many CNS active agents have been identified.

MEDICATION EFFECTS ON REM SLEEP

The original and simple model of REM sleep neurochemistry is called the reciprocal interaction model.[9] This theoretic model describes the interplay between two major neuromodulator systems (aminergic and cholinergic) involved in REM sleep generation in the brainstem. Subsequent work by the original investigators and others have led to revised versions that incorporate the effects of other neurotransmitter systems that have been shown to affect the generation of REM sleep in the brainstem. These investigators' most recent version of this once simple system, called AIM (Activation - Information - Mode), has become increasingly complex as other neurotransmitters and neuromodulators have been shown to affect REM sleep generation.[10] The systems known to affect the generation of REM sleep include the neurotransmitters, γ-aminobutyric acid (GABA), glutamate, and glycine, as well as the neuromodulators, histamine, nitric oxide, adenosine, dopamine, and other less well described neuropeptides.[10,11]

Data based on clinical trials and case reports of effects and side effects of clinically used pharmaceutical agents indicate that a different pattern of medications induces disordered dreaming and nightmares than the medications reported to affect REM sleep (**Table 1**). The medications associated with clinical reports of disordered dreaming differ from those postulated to induce nightmares based on the association of dreaming with REM sleep rebound.[5,6] Medications affecting REM sleep, such as the acetyl-cholinesterase inhibitors that increase cholinergic activity are rarely associated with clinical trial and case reports of nightmares and disordered dreaming. Medications known to suppress REM sleep, such as the various types of antidepressants and benzodiazepines, are often reported to induce disordered dreaming and nightmares. Almost all medications reported to induce daytime sleepiness as an effect or side effect are also reported to induce nightmares and disordered dreaming (**Table 2**). The neurochemistry of medication effects on dreaming seems more complex than even the modified reciprocal interaction model of REM sleep.

As discussed previously, disordered dreaming and nightmares are also commonly reported during the withdrawal from addictive medications and drugs of abuse. This finding has been postulated as secondary to the occurrence of REM sleep rebound during withdrawal from REM sleep–suppressant medication. In the case of withdrawal from REM sleep, suppressant addictive medications, such as ethanol and benzodiazepines, this explanation may be correct at least in part. Nightmares and disordered dreaming, however, are often reported as part of the withdrawal syndrome from none REM sleep-suppressant addictive medications, such as cannabis, cocaine, and opiates.[12,13] This finding suggests that disturbed dreaming and nightmares may be an intrinsic part of the process of withdrawal from addictive agents.[6]

PRIMARY NEUROTRANSMITTERS AND NEUROMODULATORS AFFECTING SLEEP AND DREAMING
Acetylcholine

Acetylcholine is the primary neuromodulator affecting REM sleep. Cholinergic agonists are most likely to increase percentages of REM sleep, with cholinergic antagonists tending to decrease REM sleep.[14,15] A wide variety of pharmaceutical agents have anticholinergic activity and the reported side effects of some of these agents include nightmares, disordered dreaming, and hallucinations. This has led some investigators to postulate that cholinergic effects of medications induce nightmares, hallucinations, and psychosis as side effects.[16] Anticholinesterase agents that increase CNS acetylcholine levels, however, are in widespread use for the treatment of the cognitive effects of Alzheimer disease. These agents are reported to induce the side effect of disturbed dreaming or nightmares in only 0.4% of clinical trial participants (see **Table 1**).

Norepinephrine

Many of the drugs in general use for treating high blood pressure (hypertension) affect norepinephrine receptors. β- and $α_1$-adrenergic antagonists have been shown to affect REM sleep and reports of dreaming. Because these agents suppress REM sleep, they are sometimes used clinically in the treatment of recurrent nightmares in patients with posttraumatic stress disorder (PTSD). Yet the norepinephrine affecting antihypertensive agents classified as β-blockers and α-agonists are responsible for 34% of clinical trials in which nightmares are reported as an adverse effect.[17] The reported effects of these agents on dreams and nightmares is often opposite to the drug's known pharmacologic effects on REM sleep. Decreases in dream recall occur with use of α-agonists (eg, minoxidil) that are REM suppressant and β-blockers (eg, propranolol and atenolol) that do not suppress REM sleep. The use of β-blockers depresses REM sleep percentages yet can result in reports of increased dreaming, nightmares, and hallucinations.[18,19] The effects of these agents demonstrate that a drug's effect on REM sleep may or may not be associated with an associated change in reported dreaming.

Serotonin

Many antidepressants exert primary effects at serotonin receptors; however, these agents also affect a variety of other neurotransmitters (see **Table 1**). Serotonin and norepinephrine are proposed to have functional roles in the production of REM sleep. Most antidepressants suppress REM sleep. This effect is greatest for the monoamine oxidase inhibitors (MAOIs) and the tricyclic antidepressants (eg, amitryptiline and imipramine). The selective serotonin reuptake inhibitors (SSRIs) (eg, paroxetine and sergeline), however, are potent supressors of REM sleep. Most antidepressants are reported in clinical trials to induce nightmares in some patients.[5,6,20] Intense visual dreaming and nightmares are associated with the acute withdrawal from some antidepressants.[21] This effect could be due to REM sleep rebound occurring after the withdrawal of these REM sleep–suppressant agents; however, studies of reported dream recall with antidepressant use show that recall may vary independently of REM sleep suppression.[22] Studies of chronic steady state use and antidepressant withdrawal have shown inconsistent effects: increased dream recall with SSRIs and tricyclics, no effect, and decreased recall.[23]

Dopamine

Dopamine receptor stimulation commonly results in the reported side effect of drug-induced nightmares. The use of dopamine, bromocriptine, pergoline, pramipexole, and other dopamine agonists can lead to vivid dreaming,

nightmares, and night terrors, which can be the first signs of the development of drug-induced psychosis.[24] Amphetamine use has been linked to nightmares (16% of nightmare reports from clinical trials). This effect has been postulated to occur secondary to dopamine receptor stimulation.[17]

γ-Aminobutyric Acid

GABA is the primary negative feedback neurotransmitter in the CNS. Almost all medications classified as hypnotics exert behavioral effects at the GABA receptor. Psychopharmacologic GABA effects extend beyond sleep and include anxiolysis, sedation, amnesia, myorelaxation, anesthesia, pain relief, tolerance, possible abuse potential, and interactions with ethanol.[25–27] These various effects are modulated at specific GABA receptor subtypes with gating properties varying markedly depending on subunit combinations.[28] Agents with general and indiscriminate effects on the GABA receptor induce a combination of effects, often with negative and detrimental consequences. The medications and drugs of abuse used to treat insomnia exert primary effects at the GABA receptor and include ethanol, barbiturates, barbiturate-like agents, and the benzodiazepines. Effects of these agents are general and indiscriminate at each of the GABA A subtypes resulting in sedative and amnesic as well as hypnotic drug effects.[29] Chronic ethanol use has been shown to alter the activity of the GABA A receptor complex.[30] This drug-induced imbalance of GABA inhibition has been proposed as a common feature characterizing ethanol, barbiturate, and benzodiazepine dependency disorders.[31] Twenty-four percent of reports of nightmares are from benzodiazepine clinical trials.[17] The newer nonbenzodiazepine hypnotics that have not been associated at clinical dosages with REM sleep suppression or REM sleep rebound on withdrawal have been reported to induce nightmares in several clinical trials as have other agents affecting GABA reuptake inhibition.[5,6] The finding that different types of drugs known to affect the GABA receptor (agonists, modulators, and reuptake inhibitors) can result in patient complaints of nightmares and abnormal dreaming is suggestive that this neurotransmitter, that is so important in the modulation of sleep, may also exert control over neuronal populations involved in dreaming.

Histamine

Case reports indicate that the commonly used antihistamine chlorpheniramine induces nightmares

Table 1
Medications reported to induce nightmares

Affected Neuroreceptor Drug	Patient Reports of Nightmares—Evidence Base = Clinical Trials, Case Reports, or Clinical Studies	Probability Assessment of Drug Effect
Acetylcholine–cholinergic agonists		
Donepezil	CT (3/747 report disordered dreaming)	Possible
Rivastigmine	CT (abnormal dreaming in 1/100–1/1000 of patients)	Possible
Norepinephrine–β-blockers		
Atenolol	CT (3/20 patients)	Probable
Bisopropol	CT (3/68 patients): CR (1)—dechallenge	Probable
Labetalol	CT (5/175 patients)	Probable
Oxprenolol	CT (11/130 patients)	Probable
Propranolol	CT (8/107 patients)	Probable
Norepinephrine effecting agents		
Guanethidine	CT (4/48 patients)	Probable
Serotonin–SSRI		
Fluoxetine	CT (1%–5%)—greater frequency in OCD and bulemic trials: CR (4)—de- and rechallenge	Probable
Escitalopram oxylate	CT (abnormal dreaming—1% of 999 patients)	Probable
Nefazodone	CT (3% [372] vs 2% control)	Probable
Paroxetine	CT (4% [392] vs 1% control)	Significant
Agents affecting serotonin and norepinephrine		
Duloxetine	CT (>1% report of nightmare/abnormal dreaming—23983 patients)	Probable
Risperidone	CT (1% increased dream activity—2607 patients)	Probable
Venlafaxine	CT (4% [1033] vs 3% control)	Probable
Agents affecting norepinephrine and dopamine		
Buproprion	CT (13/244—dream abnormality)	Probable
Norepinephrine, serotonin, and dopamine reuptake inhibitor		
Sibutramine	Postmarketing case report	Possible
Dopamine–agonists		
Amantadine	CT (5% report abnormal dreams): CR (1)	Probable
Levodopa	CT (2/9 patients)	Probable
Ropinirole	CT (3% [208] report abnormal dreaming vs 2% placebo)	Probable
Selegiline	CT (2/49 reporting vivid dreams)	Probable

Amphetamine-like agents		
Bethanidine	CT (2/44 patients)	Probable
Fenfluramine	CT (7/28 patients): CR (1) de- and rechallenge	Probable
Phenmetrazine	CT (3/81 patients)	Probable
GABA		
γ-hydroxybutyrate	CT (nightmares >1% 473 patients)	Probable
Triazolam	CT (7/21 patients)	Probable
Zopiclone	CT (3–5/83 patients)	Probable
Nicotine agonists		
Varenicline	CT (abnormal dreams 14/821 patients)	Probable
Nicotine patches	CS (disturbed dreaming in up to 12%, affects tendency to use treatment)	Probable
Anti-infectives and immunosupressants		
Amantadine	CT (5% reporting abnormal dreams): CR (1)	Probable
Fleroxacin	CT (7/84 patients)	Probable
Ganciclovir	CR (1)—de- and rechallenge	Probable
Gusperimus	CT (13/36 patients)	Probable
Antipsychotics		
Clozapine	CT (4%)	Probable
Antihistamines		
Chlorpheniramine	CT (4/80 patients)	Probable
Angiotensin-converting enzyme inhibitors		
Enalapril	CT (0.5%–1% abnormal dreaming—2987 patients)	Probable
Losartin potassium	CT (>1% dream abnormality—858 patients)	Probable
Quinapril	CT	Probable
Other agents		
Digoxin	CR (1)—de- and rechallenge	Probable
Naproxen	CR (1)—de- and rechallenge	Probable
Verapamil	CR (1)—de- and rechallenge	Probable

Medications included in each class are those considered most likely to induce nightmares based on a quantitative meta-analysis of clinical trials, clinical studies, and case reports.
Abbreviations: CR, case reports; CS, clinical study; CT, clinical trials.
Data from Pagel JF. Helfer P. Drug induced nightmares—an etiology based review. Hum Psychopharmacol 2003;18:59–67; and Pagel JF. The neuropharmacology of nightmares in "sleep and sleep disorders: neuropsychopharmacologic approach." Pandi-Perumal SR, Cardinali DP, Lander M, editors. Georgetown (TX): Landes Bioscience; 2006. p. 225–40.

Table 2
Cognitive effects and side effects of medications: neurotransmitter/neuromodulator–associated CNS effects

Basis for CNS Activity	Sleepiness	Insomnia	Alterations in Dreaming
Neuromodulator- or neurotransmitter-mediated effects			
Serotonin	+++[a]	++[b]	+++
Norepinephrine	++	++	+++
Dopamine	+++	+++	+++
Histamine	+++	+[c]	++
GABA	+++	+	++
Acetylcholine	−[d]	++	−
Adenosine	+	+++	−
Nicotine	−	+++	+++
Other medication effects			
Effects on inflammation	++	++	++
Addictive drug withdrawal	+	+++	+++
Altered conscious interaction with environment	+++	+	++
Alterations in sleep-associated disease	+++	+++	+

[a] +++, A majority of drugs with this activity cause this effect in >5% of patients.
[b] ++, Some drugs with this activity induce this effect in 1% to 5% of patients.
[c] +, An idiosyncratic effect for some agents in this group or a withdrawal effect.
[d] −, Reported in less than 1% of patients using agents affecting this neurotransmitter/neuromodulator effect.

in some patients suggesting a potential role for histamine as a modulator of dreaming. Because of the high frequency of use of over-the-counter preparations containing this medication for sleep induction and the treatment of allergies, this may be the medication most often responsible for drug-induced disordered dreaming and nightmares.

Nicotine

Nicotine affects muscarinic cholinergic receptors. Specific nicotine receptors, however, are present throughout the CNS with demonstrated regional variance and with a diversity of effects on receptor systems.[32] Nicotine is proposed to exert primary effects, including neurotoxicity on interpeduncular cholinergic neurons.[33] Clinically, nicotine contributes to hyperarousal and can induce insomnia. Transdermal nicotine patches are reported to induce abnormal dreaming.[34] In some clinical trials this effect of inducing bad dreams has been serious enough to contribute to treatment failure.[35] Varenicline, a selective α4β2 nicotinic acetylcholine receptor partial agonist approved for smoking cessation, induces abnormal dreaming in 13% and insomnia in 18% of clinical trial participants.[36]

OTHER MEDICATION TYPES REPORTED TO INDUCE SLEEP-ASSOCIATED CNS SIDE EFFECTS
Agents Affecting Host Defense

A diverse group of antibiotics, antivirals, and immunosupressant drugs can induce the complaint of sedation, insomnia, and nightmares for some patients.[37–39] An apparent interaction exists between host defense and infectious disease as well as between the cognitive effects on sleep and dreaming for these agents. A clear, but currently poorly defined, relationship exists between host defense and infectious disease and sleep/dreaming.

Anesthetics

Some of the agents reported to cause altered dreaming are induction anesthetics used in surgery. An increased incidence of pleasant dreams are reported with profolol use.[40] The barbituate thiopental, ketamine, and the opiate, tramadol, have produced disordered dreaming and nightmares.[41,42] Some of the agents associated with the complaint of nightmares also can induce waking hallucinations and confusion (fleroxacin, triazolam, ethanol withdrawal, and amphetamines). This association suggests that agents that alter an individual's conscious relationship to the external environment can alter dream and nightmare occurrence and has, in part, led to proposals that dreams and nightmares are hallucinatory experiences occurring during sleep.[43]

OTHER MEDICATIONS

Other neurotransmitter modulators proposed to affect sleep and dreaming include orexin, adenosine, glycine, glutamate, nitric acid, and neuropeptides.[11] The neurochemical and pharmacologic basis for sleep-associated cognitive side effects for the remaining agents (see **Table 1**) without noted neurotransmitter basis remains poorly defined.

OVERVIEW—THE NEUROCHEMISTRY OF COGNITIVE SLEEP-ASSOCIATED MEDICATION SIDE EFFECTS

The group of pharmacologic preparations, psychotropic and otherwise, reported to alter sleep and dreaming is extensive and diverse (see **Tables 1** and **2**). Almost all of the agents exerting their neurochemical effects on dopamine, nicotine, histamine, GABA, serotonin, and norepinephrine alter sleep and dreaming for some patients. The effects of these agents on dreaming are unassociated or opposite to the known effects of these agents on REM sleep. Based on medication effects and side-effect profiles, evidence is limited supporting the association of the neuromodulator acetylcholine with dreaming.

Other medications seem to affect sleep and dreaming by affecting an individual's conscious relationship to the environment (anesthetics) or by affecting chemical mediators involved in the inflammatory response. Most of the agents reported to alter dreaming also induce CNS side effects of daytime somnolence or insomnia. The tendency of drugs to induce the cognitive side effects of daytime sleepiness and insomnia may be an indicator for drugs likely to induce disordered dreaming and nightmares. When queried in clinical trials as to alterations in sleep-associated cognition, many patients report such side effects. Currently there is limited assessment routinely used in the assessment of drugs without a clear theoretic history of the potential for sleep-associated cognitive side effects, such as diabetic, antibiotic, host-defense, and dietary-suppressant medications. With increasing understanding of the complexity of the sleep state and its affects on multiple physiologic systems, it

seems appropriate to incorporate such assessments into studies for most if not all medications subjected to clinical trials.

The fact that a wide spectrum of pharmacologic agents is reported to induce disturbed dreaming and nightmares suggests that the biochemical basis for dreaming is more complex and less understood than generally suggested. Among prescription medications in clinical use, β-blockers affecting norepinephrine neuroreceptors are the agents most likely to result in patient complaints of disturbed dreaming. The strongest clinical evidence for a drug to induce disordered dreaming or nightmares is for the SSRI, paroxetine, a medication known to suppress REM sleep. Acetylcholinesterase inhibitors affecting the acetylcholine neuroreceptor system rarely result in patient complaints of drug-induced nightmares. Studies of drug effects and side effects do not support theoretic postulates that cholinergic neurons (the triggers for REM sleep) serve as a primary neuroreceptor system involved in dreaming and nightmares. Disturbed dreaming and nightmares are reported during withdrawal from addictive medications. This complaint occurs with drugs without known REM sleep suppression or rebound during withdrawal, suggesting that disturbance in dreaming in this situation may characterize withdrawal from addictive agents rather than being secondary to REM sleep rebound as historically postulated.

Based on its neurochemistry, dreaming does not seem to be a simple or derivative state of REM sleep. Dreaming is most likely to be affected by medications inducing effects or side effects of insomnia or daytime sleepiness and altering alertness and cognitive interaction with the world. Neurochemically, dreaming is a state of consciousness with an inherent neurochemical complexity similar to waking.

MEDICATION EFFECTS ON PARASOMNIAS

Medication-induced changes in sleep stages can lead to an increase in symptoms occurring during those specific sleep/dream states. Medications, such as lithium, opiates, and γ-hydroxybutyrate (sodium oxybate), that can cause an increase in deep sleep can induce the occurrence of arousal disorders, such as somnambulism.[44] Nicotine, caffeine, and alcohol also have been implicated in somnambulism, possibly because of their tendencies to increase nocturnal arousals.[45]

REM behavior disorder (RBD) can be triggered by a variety of antidepressant medications as well as dopamine agonists and anticholinergics used to treat Alzheimer disease. Acute RBD has been noted to occur during the withdrawal from cocaine, amphetamines, benzodiazepines, ethanol, barbiturates, and meprobamate.[46] Caffeine may unmask RBD. The influence of psychoactive medications on sleep states has a positive side as well. For example, REM sleep–suppressant medications can be useful adjuncts in the treatment of REM sleep parasomnias and other REM sleep stage–specific symptoms. Benzodiazepines and antidepressants can be used to decrease REM sleep. Similarly, the arousal disorders can be treated with medications affecting deep sleep (benzodiazepines and others). Clonazepam (Klonopin) is the medication most commonly used in the treatment of parasomnias, particularly in cases of RBD.

MEDICATIONS FOR TREATING NIGHTMARES AND PTSD

Individuals with PTSD have characteristic symptoms of recurrent nightmares and hyperarousal affecting sleep and waking. Currently, the best data demonstrate significant improvement in nightmares for cognitive-based imagery therapy.[47–49] This approach deemphasizes discussion of the traumatic association of nightmares emphasizing, instead, habitual pattern of recurrent nightmares. This approach is coupled with cognitive insomnia therapy, including sleep hygiene, stimulus control, and sleep restriction. Significant improvements have been obtained using this approach in nightmare frequency, sleep quality, anxiety, and depression.

PTSD nightmares are often treated with prolonged exposure therapy that includes focusing and reliving the traumatic experience. This approach, coupled with medication (typically SSRI antidepressants) has shown evidence for improved outcomes compared to individuals treated with medication.[50] Such critical incident stress debriefing (CISD) approaches to the treatment of PTSD are currently in general use in military and civilian first response units.[51] In the modern world, PTSD is common and psychological services have limited availability, so psychoactive medications are often used in the treatment of PTSD, even when shown to have limited efficacy.

Medications used for the treatment of PTSD run the gamut of the psychoactive pharmacopoeia. Despite limited evidence as to efficacy, the current medications recommended for the treatment of PTSD are the SSRI antidepressants.[51–53] Medications that have shown positive efficacy in case reports include antianxiety agents, nonbenzodazepine hypnotics, antidepressants, mood stabilizers, anticonvulsants, and antipsychotics.[54–61] These medications are in general use for the treatment of PTSD in children and adolescents.[58] The acute use of hypnotics after trauma does not prevent the development of PTSD.[60] Partial responders to pharmacologic treatment often require the addition of a second class of medication.[53] The effects of these agents on nightmare frequency in PTSD have not been addressed for most of these agents, except for the antidepressants, trazadone, nefazodone, and fluoxamine, which have been shown to decrease nightmare frequency and sometimes improve the insomnia associated with chronic PTSD.[53,61]

It has been postulated that some patients with PTSD exhibit abnormalities in noradrenergic function.[62] Antihypertensive agents in general use affect noradrenergic CNS receptors. These drugs have been shown to affect REM sleep and reports of dreaming. Decreases in dream recall occur with use of α-agonists (REM suppressant) and β-blockers (non-REM suppressant).[63] An agent's effect on REM sleep may or may not be associated with an associated change in reported dreaming.[5,6] β-Blockers (propranolol) have shown positive results in the treatment of PTSD despite tendencies to increase the frequency of reported nightmares.[18] Prazosin is the α-agonist most commonly used for the treatment of recurrent nightmares in PTSD patients. Significant decreases in disturbing dreams and improvement in sleep onset and maintenance insomnia have been achieved in PTSD patients.[53,64]

A meta-analysis of the literature on the pharmacotherapy of PTSD reached the conclusion that medication treatments can be useful in the treatment of PTSD and should be considered as part of the treatment of this disorder.[65] Although there was limited evidence showing that one class of medications is more effective than any other, the greatest number of trials showing efficacy to date has been with the SSRIs. In contrast, there were negative studies for benzodiazepines, MAOIs, antipsychotics, lamotrigine, and inositol. Maximizing treatment outcomes seemed to require behavioral psychotherapy in addition to medication use. Maintenance trials also suggested that long-term behavioral interventions increase the efficacy of medications and prevent relapse.[48]

SUMMARY

The sleep-associated cognitive states of dreaming are neurochemically complex. Almost all drugs affecting dopamine, nicotine, histamine, GABA, serotonin, and norepinephrine alter dreaming and reported nightmare frequency in some patients.

Other medications apparently affect sleep and dreaming by altering an individual's conscious relationship to the environment (anesthetics) or by affecting inflammatory response. Changes in reported dream and nightmare recall frequency are most clearly associated with medications that induce alterations in alertness/arousal. Medications affecting alertness with clinical cognitive effects or side effects of arousal (insomnia) or sedation commonly alter the reported frequency of dreaming and nightmares. There is good evidence that prazosin can lead to diminished nightmare frequency and improved sleep in patients with PTSD-associated nightmares. Although SSRI antidepressants are commonly used for the treatment of PTSD, evidence for efficacy is limited when compared to results attained with cognitive and behavioral approaches to treatment. These medications work best when used with appropriate behavioral therapies.

REFERENCES

1. Foulkes D. Dreaming: a cognitive-psychological analysis. Hillsdale (NJ): Lawrence Erlbaum Associates; 1985.
2. Solms M. The neurophysiology of dreams: a clinico-anatomical study. Mahwah (NJ): Lawrence Erlbaum; 1997.
3. Pagel JF. The limits of dream—a scientific exploration of the mind/brain interface. Oxford (UK): Academic Press (Elsiever); 2008.
4. Domhoff GW. The scientific study of dreams—neural networks, cognitive development, and content analysis. Washington, DC: American Psychological Association; 2003.
5. Pagel JF, Helfer P. Drug induced nightmares—an etiology based review. Hum Psychopharmacol 2003;18:59–67.
6. Pagel JF. The neuropharmacology of nightmares in "sleep and sleep disorders: neuropsychopharmacologic approach". In: Pandi-Perumal SR, Cardinali DP, Lander M, editors. Sleep and sleep disorders: a neuropsychopharmacologic approach. Georgetown (TX): Landes Bioscience; 2006. p. 225–40.
7. Kandle ER. The brain and behavior. In: Kandel ER, Schwartz JH, Jessell TM, editors. Principles of neural science. 4th edition. New York: McGraw Hill; 2000. p. 5–18.
8. Schwartz JH. Neurotransmitters. In: Kandel ER, Schwartz JH, Jessell TM, editors. Principles of neural science. 4th edition. New York: McGraw Hill; 2000. p. 280–97.
9. McCarley R, Hobson J. Neuronal excitability modulation over the sleep cycle: a structural and mathematical model. Science 1975;189:58–60.
10. Hobson J, Pace-Schott E, Stickgold R. In: Pace-Schott E, Solms M, Blagtove M, et al, editors, Dreaming and the brain: toward a cognitive neuroscience of conscious states in sleep and dreaming: scientific advances and reconsiderations 2003. p. 1–50.
11. Pace-Schott EF. Postscript: recent findings on the neurobiology of sleep and dreaming. In: Pace-Schott EF, Solms M, Blagrove M, et al, editors. Sleep and dreaming: scientific advances and reconsiderations. Cambridge (UK): Cambridge University Press; 2003. p. 335–50.
12. Bundley AJ, Hughes JR, Moore BA, et al. Marijuana abstinence effects in marijuana smokers maintained in their home environment. Arch Gen Psychiatry 2001;58(10):917–24.
13. Wade DT, Makela PM, House H, et al. Long term use of a cannabis-based medicine in the treatment of spasticity and other symptoms in multiple sclerosis. Mult Scler 2006;12(5):639–45.
14. Hobson JA, Steriade M. The neuronal basis of behavioral state control: internal regulatory systems of the brain. In: Bloom F, Mountcastle V, editors, Handbook of psychology, vol. IV. Washington, DC: American Physiological Society; 1986. p. 701–823 (14).
15. Steriade M. Brain electrical activity and sensory processing during waking and sleeping states. In: Kryger MH, Roth T, Dement WC, editors. Principles and practice of sleep medicine. 3rd edition. Philadelphia: W.B. Saunders Co; 2000. p. 93–111.
16. Perry E, Perry R. Acetylcholine and hallucinations: disease related compared to drug induced alterations in human consciousness. Brain Cogn 1995; 28:240–58.
17. Thompson D, Pierce D. Drug induced nightmares. Ann Pharmacother 1999;33:93–6.
18. Dimsdale J, Newton R. Cognitive effects of beta-blockers. J Psychosom Res 1991;36(3):229–36.
19. Brismar K, Motgensen L, Wetterberg L. Depressed melatonin secretion in patients with nightmares due to beta-adrenoceptor blocking drugs. Acta Med Scand 1987;221(2):155–8.
20. Coupland NJ, Bell CJ, Potokar JP. Serotonin reuptake inhibitor withdrawal. J Clin Psychopharmacol 1996;16(5):356–62.
21. Pace-Schott E, Gersh T, Silvestri R, et al. Effects of serotonin reuptake inhibitors (SSRI) on dreaming in normal subjects. Sleep 1999;22(Suppl 1):H278D.
22. Lepkifker E, Dannon PN, Iancu I, et al. Nightmares related to fluoxetine treatment. Clin Neuropharmacol 1995;18(1):90–4.
23. Pace-Schott E, Gersh T, Silvestri R, et al. Enhancement of subjective intensity of dream features in normal subjects by the SSRI's paroxetine and fluvoxamine. Sleep 2000;23(Suppl 2):A173.
24. Stacy M. Managing late complications of Parkinson's disease. Med Clin North Am 1999;83(2):469–81.

25. Atack J. Anxioselective compounds acting at the GABA A receptor benzodiazepine binding site. Curr Drug Targets CNS Neurol Disord 2003;2:213–32.

26. Whiting P. GABA-A receptor subtypes in the brain: a paradigm for CNS drug discovery? Drug Discov Today 2003;8:445–50.

27. Wafford K, Macaulay R, O'Meara G, et al. Differentiating the role of γ – aminobutyric acid type A (GABA A) receptor subtypes. Biochem Soc Trans 2004;32: 553–6.

28. Krogsgaard-Larsen P, Frolund B, Liljefors T. Specific GABA A agonists and partial agonists. Chem Rec 2002;2:419–30.

29. Stahl S. Selective actions on sleep or anxiety by exploiting GABA-A/benzodiazepine receptor subtypes. J Clin Psychiatry 2002;63:179–80.

30. Rassnick S, Krechman J, Koob G. Chronic ethanol produces a decreased sensitivity to the response – disruptive effects of GABA receptor complex antagonists. Pharmacol Biochem Behav 1993;44:943–50.

31. Schlosser R, Gesierich T, Wagner G, et al. Altered benzodiazepine receptor sensitivity in alcoholism: a study with fMRI and acute lorazepam challenge. Psychiatry Res 2007;154:241–51.

32. Collis S, Wade D, Londen J, et al. Neurochemical alterations produced by daily nicotine exposure in peri-adolescent versus adult rats. Eur J Pharmacol 2004;502:75–85.

33. Ciani E, Severi S, Bartesaghi R, et al. Neurochemical correlates of nicotine neurotoxicity on rat habenulo-interpedicular cholinergic neurons. Neurotoxicology 2005;26(3):467–74.

34. Smith TM, Winters FD. Smoking cessation: a clinical study of the trans dermal nicotine patch. J Am Osteopath Assoc 1995;95(11):655–6, 661–2.

35. Ivers RG, Farrington M, Burns CB, et al. A study of the use of free nicotine patches by indigenous people. Aust N Z J Public Health 2003;27(5):486–90.

36. Lam S, Patel PN. Varenicline: a selective alpha4-beta2 nicotinic acetylcholine receptor partial agonist approved for smoking cessation. Cardiol Rev 2007; 15(3):154–61.

37. Krueger JM, Fang J. Host defense. In: Kryger M, Roth T, Dement W, editors, Principles and practice of sleep medicine, vol. 3. Philadelphia: W.B. Saunders Co; 2000. p. 255–65.

38. Krueger JM, Kubillis S, Shoham S, et al. Enhancement of slow wave sleep by endotoxin and libid A. Am J Phys 1986;251:R591–7.

39. Jaffe SE. Sleep and infectious disease. In: Kryger M, Roth T, Dement W, editors, Principles and Practice of sleep medicine, vol. 3. Philadelphia: W.B. Saunders Co; 2000. p. 1093–102.

40. Marsh S, Schaefer HG, Tschau C, et al. Dreaming and anesthesia: total i.v. anaesthesia with propofol versus balanced volitile anaeshthesia with enflurane. Eur J Anaesthesiol 1992;9:331–3.

41. Krissel J, Dick WF, Leysen KH, et al. Thiopentone, thiopentone/ketamine, and ketamine for induction of anesthesia in caesarean section. Eur J Anaesthesiol 1994;11:115–22.

42. Oxorn D, Ferris LE, Harrington E, et al. The effects of midazolam on propofol-induced anesthesia: propofol dose requirements, mood profiles, and perioperative dreams. Anesth Analg 1997;85:553–9.

43. Hobson JA. Dreaming as delerium. Cambridge Mass: MIT Press; 1999.

44. Guilleminault C, Palombini L, Pelayo R, et al. Sleepwalking and sleep terrors in prepubertal children: what triggers them? Pediatrics 2003;111(1):e17–25.

45. Schenck CH, Hurwitz TD, Mahowald MW. Symposium: normal and abnormal REM sleep regulation: REM sleep behaviour disorder: an update on a series of 96 patients and a review of the world literature. J Sleep Res 1993;2(4):224–31.

46. Schenck CH, Mahowald, Parasomnias MW. Managing bizarre sleep-related behavior disorders. Postgrad Med 2000;107(3):145–56.

47. Krakow B, Kellner R, Pathak D, et al. Imagery rehearsal treatment for chronic nightmares. Behav Res Ther 1995;33(7):837–43.

48. Robertson M, Humphreys L, Ray R. Psychological treatments for posttraumatic stress disorder: recommendations for the clinician based on a review of the literature. J Psychiatr Pract 2004;10(2):106–18.

49. Krakow B, Niedhardt J. Conquering bad dreams and nightmares. New York: Berkley Books; 1992.

50. Burgess M, Gill M, Marks I. Postal self-exposure treatment of recurrent nightmares. Randomised controlled trial. Br J Psychiatry 1998;172:257–62.

51. Bisson J, Andrew M. Psychological treatment of post-traumatic stress disorder (PTSD). Cochrane Database Syst Rev 2005;(2):CD003388.

52. Putnam FW, Hulsmann JE. Pharmacotherapy for survivors of childhood trauma. Semin Clin Neuropsychiatry 2002;7(2):129–36.

53. Schoenfeld FB, Marmar CR, Neylan TC. Current concepts in pharmacotherapy for posttraumatic stress disorder. Psychiatr Serv 2004;55(5):519–31.

54. Rapaport MH, Endicott J, Clary CM. Posttraumatic stress disorder and quality of life: results across 64 weeks of sertraline treatment. J Clin Psychiatry 2002;63(1):59–65.

55. Bartzokis G, Lu PH, Turner J, et al. Adjunctive risperidone in the treatment of chronic combat-related posttraumatic stress disorder. Biol Psychiatry 2005; 57(5):474–9.

56. Douglas Bremner J, Mletzko T, Welter S, et al. Treatment of posttraumatic stress disorder with phenytoin: an open-label pilot study. J Clin Psychiatry 2004;65(11):1559–64.

57. Hamner MB, Brodrick PS, Labbate LA. Gabapentin in PTSD: a retrospective, clinical series of adjunctive therapy. Ann Clin Psychiatry 2001;13(3):141–6.

58. Wheatley M, Plant J, Reader H, et al. Clozapine treatment of adolescents with posttraumatic stress disorder and psychotic symptoms. J Clin Psychopharmacol 2004;24(2):167–73.

59. Davidson JR, Weisler RH, Butterfield MI, et al. Mirtazapine vs. placebo in posttraumatic stress disorder: a pilot trial. Biol Psychiatry 2003;53(2):188–91.

60. Mellman TA, Bustamante V, David D, et al. Hypnotic medication in the aftermath of trauma. J Clin Psychiatry 2002;63(12):1183–4.

61. Warner MD, Dorn MR, Peabody CA. Survey on the usefulness of trazodone in patients with PTSD with insomnia or nightmares. Pharmacopsychiatry 2001;34(4):128–31.

62. Southwick SM, Krystal JH, Morgan CA, et al. Abnormal noradrenergic function in posttraumatic stress disorder. Arch Gen Psychiatry 1993;50(4):266–74.

63. Danchin N, Genton P, Atlas P, et al. Comparative effects of atenolol and clonidine on polygraphically recorded sleep in hypertensive men: a randomized, double-blind, crossover study. Int J Clin Pharmacol Ther 1995;33(1):52–5.

64. Raskind MA, Peskind ER, Kanter ED, et al. Reduction of nightmares and other PTSD symptoms in combat veterans by prazosin: a placebo-controlled study. Am J Psychiatry 2003;160(2):371–3.

65. Stein DJ, Ipser JC, Seedat S. Pharmacotherapy for post traumatic stress disorder (PTSD). Cochrane Database Syst Rev 2006;(1):CD002795.

Imagery Rehearsal Therapy: Principles and Practice

Barry Krakow, MD[a],*, Antonio Zadra, PhD[b]

KEYWORDS

- Dreaming • Dream frequency • Dream content
- Nightmares • Trauma • Posttraumatic dreams

Many clinicians in sleep medicine, psychiatry, and psychology remain unaware of the suffering and distress caused by chronic nightmares. This lack of awareness extends to the therapeutic tools that effectively reduce or eliminate the problem. Many nonpharmacologic techniques have been proposed to treat posttraumatic stress disorder (PTSD)–related or idiopathic nightmares, including hypnosis, lucid dreaming, eye movement desensitization and reprocessing, desensitization, and imagery rehearsal therapy (IRT). However, only desensitization and IRT have been the objects of controlled studies, and IRT has received the most empirical support. This article highlights key principles behind this technique and the practice methods used to apply it by presenting an abridged and updated version of an earlier work.[1] Further resources are also available to readers interested in additional material on the clinical use of IRT.[2,3] For those patients in whom IRT may be impractical or counterproductive, pharmacotherapy (eg, prazosin, a central α-1 adrenoreceptor blocker) may be a useful alternative therapeutic option for PTSD-related nightmares.[4,5] Readers interested in pharmacologic approaches to nightmare treatment and the issue of drug-induced nightmares are referred to another article (See the article by J.F. Pagel elsewhere in this issue for further exploration of this topic.).

CONTROLLED TREATMENT STUDIES

In the last 20 years, IRT has been tested repeatedly in various samples and has shown efficacy in reducing nightmare distress and nightmare frequency, including maintenance of changes at long-term follow-up.[6–9] IRT effectively relieves idiopathic, recurrent, and PTSD-related forms of nightmares.[6,8,10,11] In these same studies, a relatively consistent pattern emerged of decreased psychiatric distress including anxiety, depression, or PTSD symptoms, following successful nightmare treatment. Of the several hundred participants and patients, with and without PTSD, treated in research protocols with IRT, approximately 70% reported clinically meaningful improvements in nightmare frequency. However, anecdotal observations among those individuals who reported regular use of the technique for 2 to 4 weeks indicate that significant clinical change occurred in greater than 90% of patients.

Variations exist in the application of IRT[12–17] and IRT has also been adapted for use in children suffering from nighttimes.[18,19] The distinguishing features between these variations generally revolve around the degree of exposure used during treatment sessions and/or the specific application of the technique during the sessions. This article focuses on IRT as developed by Kellner, Neidhardt, Krakow, and Hollifield at the University of New Mexico School of Medicine (1988–1999) and at the Sleep & Human Health Institute (2000 to present).

THERAPEUTIC COMPONENTS OF IRT
Current Practice

IRT can be conceptualized as a 2-component therapeutic process, each of which targets

[a] Maimonides Sleep Arts & Sciences, Ltd, Maimonides International Nightmare Treatment, Sleep & Human Health Institute, 6739 Academy NE, Suite 380, Albuquerque, NM 87109, USA
[b] Department of Psychology, Université de Montréal, CP 6128, Succursale Centre-ville, Montreal, QC H3C 3J7, Canada
* Corresponding author.
E-mail address: bkrakow@sleeptreatment.com

Sleep Med Clin 5 (2010) 289–298
doi:10.1016/j.jsmc.2010.01.004

a distinct yet overlapping problem in the nightmare sufferer. The first component is an educational/cognitive restructuring element, focused on helping the nightmare sufferer to consider their disturbing dreams as a learned sleep disorder, similar to psychophysiologic insomnia. The second component is an imagery education/training element, which teaches patients who have nightmares about the nature of human imagery and how to implement a specific set of imagery steps to decrease nightmares. IRT can be delivered individually or in groups, but for either scenario the same progression of treatment steps is offered. Follow-up time is always recommended to reassess the patient.

The first 2 sessions encourage patients to recognize the effect of nightmares on their sleep by showing them how nightmares promote learned insomnia. They are offered the view that nightmares themselves may develop as a learned behavior. The final 2 sessions engage the nightmare sufferer to learn about the human imagery system, to monitor how this system operates, to appreciate the connections between daytime imagery and dreams, and to implement the specific steps of IRT (ie, selecting a nightmare, changing the nightmare into a new dream, and rehearsing the new dream). Aspects of each of these 2 components are included in all 4 sessions, but learned sleep disorders predominates in the first 2 sessions and imagery work predominates in the last 2 sessions. An overview of the main points covered in each of these sessions is presented in **Box 1**.

Throughout the sessions, we never discount or ignore patients' perspectives on triggering incidents perceived as the cause of their nightmares. This point is especially relevant for trauma survivors with nightmares and for the meanings they associate with their disturbing dreams. Nevertheless, patients are shown how nightmares can be effectively treated without any discussion or emphasis on previous traumatic events or non–sleep-related PTSD symptoms. IRT is organized to minimize exposure therapy as an ingredient of the technique.

SESSION 1
Something to Sleep On

In our largest randomized controlled trial with PTSD patients,[20] we introduced IRT by discussing how nightmares promote insomnia. This approach serves 3 purposes. First, it immediately shows the patient that our interests are truly focused on sleep-related problems and not on trauma, current negative life events, or PTSD. Second, it creates an insightful "mini-aha" experience because most trauma survivors do not generally associate

---

Box 1
Overview of the main components in each of the 4 IRT sessions

Session 1
- Reiterating that the group will not discuss past traumatic events or traumatic content of nightmares
- Addressing treatment credibility
- How nightmares can lead to insomnia
- How nightmares pass from an acute phase to a chronic disorder
- Unsuspected benefits from having nightmares

Session 2
- Why nightmares might persist long after traumatic exposure
- What happens to symptoms of low well-being when nightmares are treated directly
- Concept of symptom substitution
- Proportion of nightmares caused by trauma versus conditioning
- Principles of general imagery and pleasant imagery
- Overcoming difficulties in the use imagery

Session 3
- Broader discussion of imagery
- Imagery as a vehicle for change
- Changing one's nightmare identity

Session 4
- IRT for nightmares
- Selecting a nightmare
- Changing the nightmare any way you wish
- Rehearsing the new dream

---

their nightmares with insomnia. Third, most patients resonate with the suffering caused by poor sleep, which validates their negative sleep experiences and thus their reasons for seeking treatment of these vexing sleep disturbances.

The current version of IRT focuses on the broader concept of poor sleep quality, including a discussion of insomnia. This also sets the stage for future discussions about sleep-disordered breathing, which the authors have found in a high rate of trauma survivors with nightmares and PTSD.[21–25] The basic elements of the discussion revolve around the following points: (1) nightmares fragment sleep; (2) sleep fragmentation causes poor sleep quality; (3) poor sleep quality is a psychological and physiologic process; (4) efforts to improve sleep quality provide maximum relief of sleep problems; and (5) treating nightmares is an important step and sometimes the best first step in treating posttraumatic sleep disturbance.

Nightmare Help and Harm

Nightmares not only cause reexperiencing, but they also initiate a cascading sequence of mental and physical hyperarousal symptoms, triggered by the threats within the disturbing dreams. These arousal symptoms represent a second symptom cluster in PTSD.[26] Following arousal, patients usually search for ways of preventing this cycle from recurring, and quite naturally they seek to avoid the trigger. In this specific sleep-related instance, trauma survivors report avoiding sleep onset at bedtime or re-onset in the middle of the night with the hope of preventing more bad dreams. Although patients may not recognize sleep avoidance as a conscious process, most nightmare sufferers resonate with the schema once they hear this sequence, which again coincides with a third symptom cluster of PTSD (avoidance).

The discussion turns to the transition process through which nightmares move from an acute phase to a chronic disorder. We use a paradigm, developed by Michael Hollifield, which helps patients recognize that soon after the trauma, they made a natural and smart choice to experience nightmares. That is, disturbing dreams, by many accounts from the empirical and theoretic literature, may serve a function of emotional adaptation to emotionally salient or traumatic events.[27-30] Early after the trauma, nightmares might help to relive the experience and remember important details that might be meaningful to the survivor; the dreams might provide useful information for emotional processing, either spontaneously through dreaming, rapid eye movement sleep, or in collaboration with a therapist; and the nightmares might serve a survival function by motivating the individual to alter a behavior or some other aspect of their lifestyle to remain out of harm's way. This process leads to the closing question, "Do these nightmares and disturbing dreams still provide any benefits, once they have lasted for so long?" We suggest that individuals reflect on this question for the next week, but most people are quick to respond in the negative. This hopefully provides them with a hint at the possibility that nightmares can take on a life of their own, which is the major focus of the next session.

SESSION 2
Persistence of Nightmares

Patients who have nightmares usually believe bad dreams are uncontrollable and from the unconscious mind; yet, most want to know why the dreams have persisted for so long. To simply state that nightmares are a learned behavior is an intriguing and provocative statement that may be met by a full range of emotions and responses. This claim must be backed up with sufficient examples to persuade the patient to stay in treatment. When queried beyond the explanations of uncontrollability or unconscious processes, some patients suggest that nightmares persist because they are a long-term consequence of trauma (ie, the trauma is still causing nightmares). Others believe that the persistence of nightmares is caused by malfunctioning or altered neurotransmitters or a genetic predisposition. Occasionally, a patient initiating treatment will raise the possibility that nightmares are a habit or a learned behavior (some even speak the phrase "broken record").

However, most patients are locked into the idea that nightmares persist because trauma or other PTSD symptoms stick in their minds. This relationship is therefore examined in a few ways in an attempt to produce cognitive restructuring. First, we discuss how nightmares might "take on a life of their own." Most patients relate to this idea, because they are unsure what provokes a disturbing dream on a specific night-to-night basis. We ask whether it seems possible that some type of psychotherapy could be directly targeted at the nightmares. Could the disturbing dreams now be functioning in some distinct manner, separate from the PTSD process?

We then work through a paradigm based on the question: "If you eliminated your disturbing dreams without influencing or treating any other aspect of your mental health, what would happen to these 4 distress symptoms: anxiety, depression, somatization, and hostility?" Most patients declare these symptoms should get worse, because nightmares must have been serving a purpose. The term "symptom substitution" is used regarding this potential downside of treating nightmares directly.

We organize the discussion of this process with the example of aggressive and violent nightmares and ask patients to suggest the types of emotions experienced during such dreams. Most suggest anger and rage, and a few mention fear, guilt, horror, or grief. We focus on anger and rage, and then ask what would happen to these feelings if a person were suddenly to stop having these nightmares. Again, patients usually state that because the anger and rage have not been released through the nightmare experience, these emotions must go somewhere else, which leads to further problems (eg, symptom substitution). When they are again asked what would happen to symptoms of anxiety, depression, somatization, and hostility following direct treatment of disturbing dreams, most patients again report that these symptoms would either worsen or remain unchanged.

Learning to Have Nightmares

This phase marks a critical turning point, because we briefly but clearly describe the results from nightmare treatment research in which anxiety and other distress symptoms usually decrease after nightmares have been treated. Most patients sit back to regroup, because these results do not resonate with what they learned or believed about nightmares. Although many patients will not fully or immediately process the ramifications of this information, most participants become curious and excited about this new perspective.

In the final phase of this discussion, the patient is offered an opportunity to estimate the extent to which disturbing dreams can be attributed to trauma (0%–100%) or to habit (0%–100%) with the sum of the 2 estimates equaling 100%. Although this exercise can be performed earlier and later in the treatment, it is useful at this point because the patients have begun to experience some flux in their perceptions about why they still have nightmares.

Many telltale indicators of treatment interest or resistance arise from these estimates. Rarely, a few individuals who believe strongly that the nightmares are deeply entrenched in their trauma process will deny any habit component. Conversely, others who have completed successful psychotherapy for their traumatic exposure or other mental health problems might declare their bad dreams must be 100% habit. The former group tends to be reluctant to attempt IRT and should probably be discouraged from doing so until some shift in their views occurs in the remaining sessions. The latter group is not only ready to try IRT but these individuals may report decreases in their nightmares following this session before having learned the full IRT technique. Most individuals lie between these extremes (80–20, 50–50, or 20–80 splits are all common), but what is most interesting and informative is that nearly all of them report some shift in their perceptions toward habit recognition compared with what they would have estimated beforehand.

Imagery Skills

The discussion now focuses on imagery, which is a well-described behavioral therapy component in the treatment of many other types of medical and psychological conditions.[31] The relevant and self-explanatory elements that are discussed include (1) imagery is a natural part of mental activity, which is easily described in behavioral terms as 1 component of the mental system of thoughts, feelings, and images; (2) imagery is often the last conscious activity just before sleep onset; (3) ergo, imagery during the day may be a bridge to imagery at night (dreams); (4) imagery is not meditation but simply a daydream with bit more intention or structure as needed or desired; (5) imagery skills can be tested in brief exercises of a few minutes, and most trauma survivors have a reasonable ability to conduct such tests in groups or individually; (6) some trauma survivors are surprised at their healthy capacity to image things; and (7) most PTSD patients, except those of extreme severity, can practice pleasant imagery exercises at home without much difficulty.

Special attention is needed during this part of the session for the minority of patients with clear-cut imagery deficiencies. They may report either outright difficulty as a black or blank screen, or unpleasant images that force them to open their eyes and terminate the imagery session. All individuals are provided with behavioral tips on how to overcome unpleasant imagery (see list of common treatment obstacles in **Box 2**), but we focus on acknowledging the unpleasant image and choosing to move on to a new, preferably more pleasant or neutral image. This process is stated in the context of the thoughts, feelings, images paradigm, in which the patient appreciates the natural flux in this system. That is, the mind-body is continuously presented with new thoughts, feelings and images, and when we become aware of certain ones, we may choose to let go as we observe new ones emerging.

All patients are directed to practice pleasant imagery every day for a few minutes. The first step in this exercise is to encourage patients to recognize that imagery is a frequently experienced pathway that normal sleepers often report at sleep onset.[32,33] Conversely, nightmare sufferers may want to improve their imagery skills but without over stimulating themselves for fear of triggering more disturbing images. Although few patients report changes in their nightmares after using pleasant imagery during the ensuing week, their prospects remain high for future use of IRT because they experienced some perceived benefits from simple imagery exercises.

Imagery Practice

To practice pleasant imagery, we use 3 possible versions of standard instructions based on times of 1, 5, or 15 minutes and guided or unguided

---

Box 2
Commonly reported obstacles to treatment

1. Recurring nightmares

Patients seem to attach more meaning or intensity to recurring dreams and wonder whether IRT can work on these nightmares. These patients should be encouraged to avoid working with recurring dreams at first because they usually have more replay-like qualities, and therefore the patient is much more likely to associate the dream with specific traumatic experiences.

2. Multiple nightmares

Patients suffering from multiple different nightmares often imagine that IRT somehow must be used on each and every one of them. It often helps to explain that nightmares often exhibit similar characteristics or overlapping themes. Therefore, IRT can still be used by working on only 1 or 2 nightmares per week.

3. Feeling uncomfortable or anxious while considering a nightmare

Although patients may find it unpleasant to consider their nightmare, they should bear in mind that they only have to do it once. After they changed it into a new dream, they no longer have to work with the original nightmare.

4. Difficulty in reviewing a vague nightmare

Because IRT focuses on constructing a new dream, remembering even a small fragment of a nightmare is often sufficient to make the transition towards a new dream.

5. Not knowing how to change the nightmare

There is no single right way to change the nightmare to create the new dream. It is the patient's decision to change it any way they wish. If they are not satisfied with the new dream, it can be changed again.

6. Letting distractions get in the way

Because imagery work requires a safe, comfortable, and distraction-free environment, patients must do whatever is needed to find the quiet uninterrupted time necessary for the treatment. If one is pressed for time, then simply practice for a few minutes to keep the skill fresh in mind. Even 1 minute per day can prove sufficient.

7. Difficulty managing negative images

Most people can naturally image or learn to imagine pleasant scenes, but one should not hesitate to work with a therapist to build this skill, if needed. Focusing on positive images and not replaying negative ones is an important part of improving overall health, including more restful sleep, positive dream imagery, and more relaxed daytime functioning. The following 6 strategies can be used to manage unpleasant images: (1) stopping: clap hands while saying "Stop!"; (2) breathing: breathe in deeply and exhale the image away; (3) grounding: open eyes, feet on floor, focus on environment; (4) talking: talk to a friend or family member about images; (5) writing: write down images; (6) acknowledging and choosing: without accepting or denying, acknowledge the unpleasant image, then choose to return to a preferred image.

---

instructions, depending on the individual's needs. Some patients are nervous about imagery, whereas others have previously experienced imagery exercises. All patients start well with a 1-minute session. Most perform so well with 1 minute of imagery, no further practice is needed, and the patients can be given instructions to practice for 5 to 20 minutes per day at home. The average patient uses an imagery session of between 5 and 10 minutes.

The most prevalent barrier includes either difficulty imaging or unpleasant images. The discussion turns to managing unpleasant images or how to promote greater ease in generating pleasant images. The latter issue is dispatched by stating that most people require time to learn how to comfortably generate pleasant images, but the interval is usually measured in weeks for most nightmare sufferers, compared with months for patients with more complex PTSD. Unpleasant imagery is a more difficult issue. Once trauma survivors recognize the potential importance of imagery in the mind's eye, most will find it straightforward to acknowledge unpleasant images and then choose to let them go as new images emerge.

A rare or occasional patient will clearly demonstrate they are stuck at this point in the process. These individuals often fit with the pattern described in recent research[34–36] in which nightmares are reportedly identical to the patients' traumatic experience. As such, they tend to obsess about this relationship and often declare they cannot image anything because it will only bring up the memory of the trauma or the nightmare, which to them feels like the same thing. We caution these patients to take a step back from the program and work with their therapist on general imagery exercises if they are comfortable doing so.

Imagery Safeguards

The session concludes with the following points and reminders: (1) PTSD patients may need to stop any type of therapy that stimulates unpleasant imagery; (2) activation of the imagery system must proceed slowly and gently; (3) know your limits and know how to overcome unpleasant images; (4) learn to appreciate that some unpleasant images emerge through learned behaviors (like nightmares), as opposed to viewing all negative imagery as a direct result of stress-related processes. The final instruction is to repeat the importance of practicing pleasant imagery by selecting pleasant experiences or scenarios from one's life.

SESSION 3
Imagery in the Process of Change

The third session begins with a broader discussion of imagery to explain that many people suffering from disturbing dreams develop an imbalance in their thoughts, feelings, imagery system. As a common example, a person might think too much and spend less time with their feelings and images because the latter are more unpleasant and less manageable. A constant barrage of nightmares or disturbing waking images (eg, traumatic memories) could easily lead someone to think too much as a natural self-protective mechanism. This imbalance, however, diminishes or distorts the nightmare sufferer's natural capacity to work with his or her imagery system. Our first exercise in this third session is to show nightmare patients how important and useful imagery is in everyday life and particularly in the process of change.

The exercise begins with each participant recalling a change in his or her life that took place in the past year. The most common examples include moving to a new home or apartment, starting a new relationship, ending a relationship, entering psychotherapy, starting a new educational program, and beginning a new job. We then discuss the role of imagery involved in the

change process. Then, 3 questions are asked. In the case of someone having changed employment, the questions would be: (1) when did you actually switch jobs; (2) when did you first think about switching jobs; and (3) when did you first picture the possibility of switching jobs?

In nearly every example provided, patients remark that each of these dates preceded the last one, such that they can recall that a picture may have formed in their mind about the possibility of switching jobs long before they spent time actively thinking about this occurrence. This point is impressive. Not only do the patients learn to appreciate that imagery is a useful and valuable tool in the process of change, but they are now introduced to the concept of rehearsal. Specifically, imagery rehearsal is something that humans engage in all the time as they practice anticipated behaviors or experiences by imagining themselves in various new or old situations to see how they could behave.

Rehearsing Change with Imagery

With this backdrop, each person is asked to select something in their life they would wish to change, but specific directions are given to choose something positive or neutral to work on that will not elicit unpleasant feelings. The most commonly used example is remodeling or rearranging a particular room in the home. Each individual then undergoes a 5- to 10-minute exercise in which they picture any components they wish to reflect on in their suggested change. These imagery experiences are subsequently discussed, and the images are almost always described as positive or pleasant. Even though the exercise is conducted in the spirit of learning imagery rehearsal in the context of change, the patients are cautioned that the exercise is not conducted to foster change on whatever theme was selected. Nonetheless, routinely 10% to 50% of individuals will report the following week that they made some effort to change something related to what they had rehearsed (eg, rearranging furniture).

Nightmare Sufferer Identity

This positive exercise extends the discussion of change in the context of imagery processes and how one might see oneself before and after change. The term used here is "identity," and the discussion revolves around how nightmare sufferers usually see themselves as intractably afflicted. They have developed a nightmare sufferer identity. The point illustrates how this identity often becomes entrenched in ways not dissimilar to cigarette smokers who see themselves as smokers and incapable of changing this behavior. In discussing the problem of quitting smoking, patients accept the idea that a major barrier to change is holding onto the belief that one's identity is fixed, as in once a smoker, always a smoker. Therefore, behavioral change often benefits by finding a way to imagine the potential for a new identity (eg, a nonsmoker). With time, this type of imagery rehearsal can help smokers change identities because they have rehearsed it sufficiently to become more comfortable with their new ways of behaving.

To some, this process can provoke anxiety or fear because changing an identity might feel like they are killing off a part of themselves. Yet changes occur all the time, and through imagery practice, consciously or otherwise, humans naturally learn to appreciate these changes in identity and develop new behavioral patterns. As much as these nightmare sufferers would like to change to the identity of a good dreamer, we spend time discussing (1) how entrenched the nightmare sufferer identity might be, (2) how it would seem unfamiliar to them to not experience disturbing dreams, and (3) how imagery can help them transition to a new identity that is no longer plagued by nightmares.

The whole lesson eventually funnels into a final question: "Are you ready to let go of your nightmares?" We quickly point out that no right or wrong answer is required of such a question, but that it might be worth reflecting on in light of how one gauges one's own identity as a nightmare sufferer. Assessing how deeply the nightmare identity might be entrenched proves useful to most nightmare sufferers before they implement the full IRT technique.

The session ends on an upbeat note by asking the participants to spend the week reflecting on the possibility of becoming a dreamer with a capacity to experience more pleasant dreams instead of nightmares. They are also instructed to continue imagery practice, either their original version of pleasant imagery or a continuation of the imagery as a vehicle for the change concept developed in this session.

SESSION 4

The fourth session uses Neidhardt's variation to "change the nightmare anyway you wish,"[8,37] but we no longer suggest that the patient write down the old nightmare unless such a process is helpful in learning the technique. The full instructions involve the following: (1) select a disturbing dream, preferably 1 of lesser intensity and not a reenactment of a trauma; (2) change this nightmare anyway you wish; (3) rehearse this new dream a few minutes each day at a time of your choosing; and (4) continue these instructions every day and consider working with another nightmare to change it into a new dream every 3 to 7 days, such that you only rehearse 1 or 2 new dreams each week.[10]

Selecting a Nightmare

How patients select their nightmares for IRT will often present clues as to how they will embrace or avoid IRT and whether or not they view it as a credible therapy. Using a crawl before you walk metaphor, we explain that IRT may have potential efficacy for all types of nightmares, but it is important to learn the technique first on disturbing dreams of lesser emotional intensity. Our goal is to trigger minimal or no emotional response as the objective is not to expose patients to traumatic content but rather to have them select a bad dream so they have material with which to learn the process of IRT. Using a replicative-trauma nightmare is therefore discouraged during first efforts.

Patients who follow the instructions to select a less threatening nightmare often find it easy to image a changed version and almost invariably find the technique palatable. In more than half of the patients with whom we have worked, it seems apparent within 15 to 30 seconds that the instruction to change the nightmare was a welcome idea, which they had probably wondered about on their own. These individuals may write down a new dream immediately for use in the rehearsal process, almost as if permission to change their dreams had finally been granted.

Changing the Nightmare

The instruction to change the nightmare sometimes meets with mild resistance primarily because of confusion with the instruction. Rarely, a patient who has nightmares may resist by declaring that changing the dream "can't be done because that's what happened to me" or "that was my dream, how can I change it?" The changes can take many forms; we are not aware of any particular change schema that is more efficacious than others, although in our experience we suspect that Neidhardt's model[8,37] to "change it anyway that feels right to you" is more powerful than narrowing the scope by suggesting to change the nightmare to something positive or triumphal. We speculate that Neidhardt's broader instruction leaves open a psychological window through which the patient may intuitively glimpse multilayered solutions to other emotional conflicts in addition to or arguably as part of their nightmare resolution. For these reasons, we remain highly suspect of techniques in which therapists or other members of a group treatment seek to impose or just suggest changes in the dream content. In our view, such an approach seems less empowering to the individual. Some patients change minutiae in the dream, whereas others develop a brand new story. In our view, it would not be surprising if an important active ingredient of IRT were shown to be the ability to reconnect with the natural human capacity to manipulate and change imagery in the mind's eye, beyond the specific changes of content within the new dreams.

Rehearsing the Nightmare

The most important instruction to give before rehearsing the dream is to remind patients they will now rehearse the new dream only and not the nightmare. In other words, we maintain our efforts at avoiding exposure and encourage patients to reinvigorate their natural capacity for imagery. This part of the session can last 5 to 15 minutes depending on the patient's comfort level and capacity for imagery. Before initiating actual IRT for nightmare treatment, patients are also reinforced with imagery training as described in session 3 to prepare them to intervene if unpleasant images arise.

Practice

Patients are informed that they are learning how to activate their imagery system in a specific way to take control of their nightmares. The early emphasis should thus be on understanding what it means to activate one's imagery system and gaining some control and comfort with that process. In time, more nightmares can be targeted if necessary, but each nightmare does not have to be subjected to imagery because IRT seems to jump start a natural human healing system that was previously dormant. In other words, working on just a few disturbing dreams and turning them into new dreams has a ripple effect on the treatment of other nightmares. The actual amount of time needed to work on any particular nightmare is variable and unpredictable, and obsessing about a particular bad dream may prove counterproductive early in treatment. Then again, we know of some patients who enjoyed and benefited from working on just 1 or 2 new dreams by constantly changing them for several months before considering any other nightmares, if any persisted. Patients learn that the program's most important step is to learn the technique and gain control and comfort with; and this effort may explain individual variation in IRT application.

At the conclusion of this session, 2 important ideas are developed to promote positive practice. First, we revisit the discussion on the relationship between dreams and imagery and talk in terms of a metamorphosis in which nightmares spontaneously change in some patients. In this view, nightmares can change early after their onset, and close inspection of the traumatic dream's content almost invariably demonstrates various alterations in detail or changes in the overall picture. This point is especially important for those patients who are stuck with the belief that their nightmares are a perfect replay of a specific event. If, over time, they can appreciate the possibility that their replays already contain altered elements, they have a reasonable chance of using IRT.

We then explain that most people with nightmares following trauma eventually stop having them. One possibility for this shift is that over a few weeks to a few months, the nightmares gradually keep changing as if the dreams themselves were working out some aspect of the emotional turmoil generated by the trauma.[27] It may therefore be natural for nightmares to surface and then gradually change into dreams that become increasingly less disturbing. The use of IRT may reflect a system similar to the natural process of mental imagery already in use in people's minds. This natural process, however, was not activated in an effective manner in these trauma patients, but IRT can now start that process.

The session is then brought to a close by reiterating the importance of working on only 1 or 2 bad dreams each week given the immediate goal of improving one's imagery system. If IRT is a naturally occurring process within the human mind, then we can argue that once the corrupted software that damaged this innate operating system is replaced, then the individual's original system can resume functioning normally. As this process unfolds, the readoption of one's natural imagery capacity may partly account for how or why patients do not need to work on each and every nightmare they experience for the treatment to be effective.

SUMMARY AND FUTURE DIRECTIONS

IRT is a proven and cost-effective therapy for chronic traumatic and idiopathic nightmares. Reduction in daytime distress following the use of IRT is consistent with the view that the direct treatment of nightmares is a feasible and worthwhile clinical approach. Clinicians' appreciation for the 2 primary therapeutic elements described in this paper should aid them in their regular use of IRT with patients experiencing nightmares. In contrast to the more rigid application of IRT in research trials, treatments in clinical settings can be provided in groups and individually and the technique shortened or lengthened to accommodate the complexity and severity of the nightmare disorder. Similarly, given the importance of the imagery component in IRT for nightmares, individuals with relatively healthy or more readily accessible imagery systems may benefit from a shortened treatment delivered on an individual or even self-help basis. Some resources have been developed for such purposes.[38,39]

IRT is an effective and versatile treatment that can alleviate various forms of nightmares and associated distress. The proper reactivation of a patient's dysfunctional imagery system and associated increase in perceived mastery over negative dream elements seem to play a vital role in nightmare reduction.

REFERENCES

1. Krakow B, Zadra A. Clinical management of chronic nightmares: imagery rehearsal therapy. Behav Sleep Med 2006;4(1):45–70.
2. Maimonides International Nightmare Treatment Center. Available at: http://www.nightmaretreatment. com/. Accessed October 26, 2009.
3. Davis JL. Treating post-trauma nightmares: a cognitive behavioral approach. New York: Springer; 2008.
4. Raskind MA, Peskind ER, Kanter ED, et al. Reduction of nightmares and other PTSD symptoms in combat veterans by prazosin: a placebo-controlled study. Am J Psychiatry 2003;160(2):371–3.
5. Taylor FB, Martin P, Thompson C, et al. Prazosin effects on objective sleep measures and clinical symptoms in civilian trauma posttraumatic stress disorder: a placebo-controlled study. Biol Psychiatry 2008;63(6):629–32.
6. Kellner R, Neidhardt J, Krakow B, et al. Changes in chronic nightmares after one session of desensitization or rehearsal instructions. Am J Psychiatry 1992; 149(5):659–63.
7. Krakow B, Kellner R, Neidhardt J, et al. Imagery rehearsal treatment of chronic nightmares: with a thirty month follow-up. J Behav Ther Exp Psychiatry 1993;24(4):325–30.
8. Neidhardt EJ, Krakow B, Kellner R, et al. The beneficial effects of one treatment session and recording of nightmares on chronic nightmare sufferers. Sleep 1992;15(5):470–3.
9. Krakow B, Kellner R, Pathak D, et al. Long term reduction of nightmares with imagery rehearsal treatment. Behav Cogn Psychother 1996;24(2):135–48.
10. Krakow B, Kellner R, Pathak D, et al. Imagery rehearsal treatment for chronic nightmares. Behav Res Ther 1995;33(7):837–43.
11. Krakow B, Tandberg D, Scriggins L, et al. A controlled comparison of self-rated sleep complaints in acute and chronic nightmare sufferers. J Nerv Ment Dis 1995;183(10):623–7.
12. Bishay N. Therapeutic manipulation of nightmares and the management of neurosis. Br J Psychiatry 1985;147:67–70.
13. Forbes D, Phelps A, McHugh T. Treatment of combat-related nightmares using imagery rehearsal: a pilot study. J Trauma Stress 2001;14(2):433–42.
14. Marks I. Rehearsal relief of a nightmare. Br J Psychiatry 1978;133:461–5.
15. Thompson JA, Charlton PF, Kerry R, et al. An open trial of exposure therapy based on deconditioning for post-traumatic stress disorder. J Clin Psychol 1995;34:407–16.
16. Lu M, Wagner A, Van ML, et al. Imagery rehearsal therapy for posttraumatic nightmares in U.S. veterans. J Trauma Stress 2009;22:236–9.
17. Germain A, Nielsen T. Impact of imagery rehearsal treatment on distressing dreams, psychological distress, and sleep parameters in nightmare patients. Behav Sleep Med 2003;1(3):140–54.
18. St-Onge MP, De Koninck J. Imagery rehearsal therapy for frequent nightmares in children. Behav Sleep Med 2009;7:81–9.
19. Simard V, Nielsen T. Adaptation of imagery rehearsal therapy for nightmares in children: a brief report. Psychotherapy: Theory, Research, Practice, Training, in press.
20. Krakow B, Hollifield M, Johnston L, et al. Imagery rehearsal therapy for chronic nightmares in sexual assault survivors with posttraumatic stress disorder: a randomized controlled trial. JAMA 2001;286(5): 537–45.
21. Krakow B, Germain A, Tandberg D, et al. Sleep breathing and sleep movement disorders masquerading as insomnia in sexual-assault survivors. Compr Psychiatry 2000;41(1):49–56.
22. Krakow B, Germain A, Warner TD, et al. The relationship of sleep quality and posttraumatic stress to potential sleep disorders in sexual assault survivors with nightmares, insomnia, and PTSD. J Trauma Stress 2001;14(4):647–65.
23. Krakow B, Melendrez D, Warner TD, et al. To breathe, perchance to sleep: sleep-disordered breathing and chronic insomnia among trauma survivors. Sleep Breath 2002;6(4):189–202.
24. Krakow B, Melendrez D, Pedersen B, et al. Complex insomnia: insomnia and sleep-disordered breathing in a consecutive series of crime victims

with nightmares and PTSD. Biol Psychiatry 2001; 49(11):948–53.

25. Krakow B, Lowry C, Germain A, et al. A retrospective study on improvements in nightmares and post-traumatic stress disorder following treatment for co-morbid sleep-disordered breathing. J Psychosom Res 2000;49(5):291–8.

26. American Psychiatric Association. Diagnostic and statistical manual of mental disorders. Text Revision (DMS-IV-TR). 4th edition. Washington, DC: APA; 2000.

27. Barrett D, editor. Trauma and dreams. Cambridge: Harvard University Press; 1996.

28. Levin R, Nielsen TA. Disturbed dreaming, posttraumatic stress disorder, and affect distress: a review and neurocognitive model. Psychol Bull 2007; 133(3):482–528.

29. Hartmann E. Dreams and nightmares: the new theory on the origin and meaning of dreams. New York: Plenum; 1998.

30. Punamaki R-L, Ali KJ, Ismahil KH, et al. Trauma, dreaming, and psychological distress among Kurdish children. Dreaming 2005;15(3):178–94.

31. Menzies V, Gill Taylor A. The idea of imagination: an analysis of "imagery". Adv Mind Body Med 2004;20: 4–10.

32. Nelson J, Harvey AG. An exploration of pre-sleep cognitive activity in insomnia: imagery and verbal thought. Br J Clin Psychol 2003;42: 271–88.

33. Nelson J, Harvey AG. Pre-sleep imagery under the microscope: a comparison of patients with insomnia and good sleepers. Behav Res Ther 2003;41:273–84.

34. Rothbaum BO, Mellman TA. Dreams and exposure therapy in PTSD. J Trauma Stress 2001; 14(3):481–90.

35. Mellman TA, David D, Bustamante V, et al. Dreams in the acute aftermath of trauma and their relationship to PTSD. J Trauma Stress 2001;14(1):241–7.

36. Mellman TA, Pigeon WR. Dreams and nightmares in posttraumatic stress disorder. In: Kryger M, Roth N, Dement WC, editors. Principles and practice of sleep medicine. 4th edition. Philadelphia: W.B. Saunders; 2005. p. 573–8.

37. Krakow B, Neidhardt EJ. Conquering bad dreams & nightmares: a guide to understanding, interpretation, and cure. New York: Berkley Books; 1992.

38. Burgess M, Gill M, Marks I. Postal self-exposure treatment of recurrent nightmares: randomised controlled trial. Br J Psychiatry 1998;172:257–62.

39. Krakow B, Krakow JK. Turning nightmares into dreams. Albuquerque: The New Sleepy Times; 2002. Available at: http://www.nightmaretreatment.com. Accessed February 1, 2010.

Dream Interpretation in Clinical Practice: A Century After Freud

Alan B. Siegel, PhD

KEYWORDS

- Dreams • Nightmares • Dream interpretation
- Psychotherapy • Posttraumatic nightmares
- Dream themes • Dream symbols

The therapeutic use of dreams was almost synonymous with the practice of psychotherapy in the twentieth century. Dream work was touted as the royal road to the unconscious and recommended as an effective vehicle for accessing hidden conflicts, enhancing the collaborative alliance, and facilitating important insights. More than a century after Freud's groundbreaking book, *The Interpretation of Dreams*,[1] some elements of his clinical theories and techniques have stood the test of time, including the use of free association, dream mechanisms (such as reversal, displacement, and condensation), and the idea that dreams reveal deeper feelings, unconscious conflicts, and past trauma. However, subsequent discoveries burst the boundaries of Freud's early wish fulfillment model. These breakthroughs included (1) the discovery of rapid eye movement (REM) in 1953, which identified the cyclic nature of dreams and allowed reliable laboratory collection of dreams; (2) more than a half century of using content analysis of dream narratives to study personality and psychopathology[2]; (3) expansion of knowledge about the functions of dreams[3]; and (4) the evolution of changes in dreaming patterns from childhood through the stages of adult development.[4] Finally, a century of case studies from various schools of psychology, such as psychoanalytic, Jungian, existential, cognitive, and humanistic, have tested innovative models and techniques with hundreds of thousands of psychotherapy patients.[5–7] This article discusses what has been learnt about how dreams can be used in psychotherapy and assessment and reviews practice guidelines for using dreams in a manner that is therapeutically effective, is within ethical guidelines, and is sensitive to cultural differences.

A METAPHORIC MODEL OF DREAM INTERPRETATION

The search for a true and objective meaning of a dream is a tantalizing goal for psychotherapists and for the lay dreamer. A brilliant interpretation satisfies the patient's hunger for reassurance, guidance, and security and fulfills the therapist's need to be helpful, knowledgeable, and effective. However, many psychotherapists do not go beyond literal interpretations of the manifest content to delve further into the metaphoric meanings of a dream. Dream and symbol dictionaries epitomize the belief that symbols have specific meanings that can instantly be decoded just by knowing what the symbols mean. The often quoted joke that "sometimes a cigar is just a cigar," implies that most of the time a cigar is actually a phallic symbol. Contemporary psychoanalytic practitioners do not interpret dreams in such a concrete and reductive manner and go beyond sex and aggression as the primary instinctual forces motivating dreams. However, in the quest for a universal model of dream interpretation, Freud's early writings may have inadvertently reinforced the notion that dream symbols have objective meanings that can only be decoded in therapy by an expert psychoanalyst.

Freud established the terms manifest and latent content to emphasize his conceptualization that the overt story, characters, symbols, and settings

Department of Psychology, University of California, Berkeley, 2607 Alcatraz Avenue, Berkeley, CA 94705, USA
E-mail address: alansiegelphd@gmail.com

Sleep Med Clin 5 (2010) 299–313
doi:10.1016/j.jsmc.2010.01.001

in a dream were a disguise for underlying meanings related to early developmental trauma. Erik Erikson[8] reanalyzed one of Freud's most renowned dreams, the Irma Dream. He established that the manifest content is a disguise and is filled with rich and psychologically meaningful symbolism. Louis Breger[9] further clarified the concept of latent content and asserted that there is no single latent content behind the camouflage of the manifest content but that there are many different possible latent meanings to any dream.

An objective or literal interpretation of a dream takes the message in the manifest content and directly links it to conflicts, feelings, or relationship dynamics that may restate conscious ideas or hunches or predict future events. This is the most frequent way that people understand and interpret dreams. For example, a dream of a plane crash may be interpreted as a warning not to fly. If thunderstorms are predicted for an upcoming flight or if you are flying on an airline with a poor safety record or on an old plane in a less-developed country, the objective meaning of such a dream may be an affirmation of an appropriate sense of fear or caution.

For those who view dreams as predictive, warning dreams that seem to be confirmed by later waking events make metaphoric interpretation seem less necessary. Thus, once you protect yourself after having a plane crash or earthquake dream, there is less urgency to consider whether a plane crash represents a loss of control or an emotional crash or whether an earthquake symbolizes a powerful inner upheaval. This becomes even more problematic with dreams that seem to predict illness, injury, or death. These dreams may strike terror in the hearts of people who believe in the inevitability of predictive dreams or intense guilt in those who believe themselves to be responsible for a tragic event that seemed to have been predicted by a dream.

Are these warning dreams intrapsychic phenomena that are most likely explained by coincidence (we know that many people dream of earthquakes and plane and car crashes every night)? Or, are they heightened intuition amplified by the dream's ability to bring together hunches and impressions? Perhaps our dreams are a sixth sense that gives us a survival mechanism to prepare for waking threats? Maybe dreams are a divine warning to be taken seriously. These are all widely held beliefs about the nature of dreams, and it is important for psychotherapists to clarify their own views and to inquire about their patient's cultural and metaphysical beliefs about the nature of dreams, especially with respect to literal interpretations.

When we intuitively sense possible danger, nightmares may serve as a survival function by warning us of imminent danger. Sleep research pioneer, William Dement, was a heavy smoker as a young adult. He reported having a dream in which a colleague was showing him radiographs of spots on his lungs with clear indications of lung cancer. The dream was so graphic and convincing that he immediately stopped smoking permanently. This is a clear example of how a literal interpretation of a dream led to a dramatic and healthy change.[10]

In a metaphoric approach to dream interpretation, investigating the possible objective meanings of a dream is only one step in the exploration and interpretive process. In addition to possibly symbolizing loss of control, a plane crash dream may suggest reconsideration of travel plans. A dream of an extramarital affair may open up a discussion of conflicts or attractions that could threaten a marriage. A dream of seeing oneself in a coffin may suggest suicidal thoughts or fears of death. These issues are important and may have been fully or partly repressed from the dreamer's conscious awareness. In that regard, sharing and exploring the dream narrative can provide a vehicle that circumvents defenses and may lead to productive consideration of pressing conflicts.

One of the author's patients, Stephen, was thoroughly puzzled by an upsetting short dream with an image of having his cash-stuffed wallet stolen by faceless thugs. Free associations about a loss of money led him to connect the wallet theft image to his painful losses in the recent stock market crash. This led to a discussion of the effect of his economic woes, a topic that had not been a prior focus of discussion. This objective and transparent linkage of being robbed in his dream opened up a valuable topic that had not been discussed previously and seemed to be connected to his symptoms of depression. This case is an example of the potential value of looking at the objective and the nearly literal level of dream interpretation.

Dreaming about losing a wallet or purse is a common theme that often symbolizes issues related to identity, to a loss of nonmonetary resources, and to stress related to finances. After delving into Stephen's associations and insights about his financial reverses, the author suggested to look at metaphors suggested by the wallet theft and mentioned the possible connection to identity issues. This idea resonated with Stephen, and he talked extensively about recent events that had transformed his identity and left him depressed. His youngest daughter had recently left for a college far from home, his wife had returned to full-time work, and he had stepped down from an active role on the board of a nonprofit group that had been the source of his self-esteem and a main avenue for his social life. The discussion of the dream also triggered a long-forgotten traumatic memory of being robbed off his wallet at gunpoint 20 years earlier and other memories about getting his first wallet when he got a summer job when he was 15 years old. For Stephen, the objective and literal link between his wallet theft dream and loss of assets led to a topic that had not been explored and related to his diminished net worth. However, exploration of the metaphoric meanings of the wallet as a painful loss and as a shift in identity opened up more sensitive topics for discussion. When he was robbed decades earlier, he was not physically injured or harmed financially and was able to cancel his credit cards and he lost only the cash in his wallet. However, the emotional trauma of that near-death experience made the dream image salient as a symbol of his current identity transformation and depression.

Dream interpretation is enriched when multiple dimensions of the meaning are considered, including what seem to be overt messages in the manifest content as well as additional layers of metaphoric meanings discovered through dialog between the dreamer and the therapist. Interpretations that seek only 1 meaning, dictated by an expert and shaped to fit a theory, are likely to be premature, reductive, and overly influenced by the biases of the therapist. The therapeutic and creative benefits of dream work come through the process of free association, collaborative exploration, and hypothesis testing, leading to insight, emotional integration, and a greater sense of meaning.

UNIVERSAL DREAMS: ASSOCIATE GLOBALLY BUT INTERPRET LOCALLY

The existence of universal symbols and themes that recur across cultures and centuries is another factor that tempts psychotherapists to rely on a dream-dictionary style of interpreting dream symbols. The reasoning is that universal dreams must surely have universal interpretations. These universal dream themes include flying, falling, paralysis, being unprepared for an examination, appearing naked in public, being chased, natural disasters, losing the wallet or purse, sexual interactions, finding new rooms in houses, mortal threats or injuries to self or others, and plane and car crashes. Although it can be helpful to know the common meanings of universal dreams, rote

interpretation of dream themes without consideration of individual differences can be misguided.

Exploring and interpreting in the light of the dreamer's unique life experience, identity, and developmental stage is especially crucial, given the lack of consensus about how to interpret dream symbols and images. Even for psychotherapists who are devoted to a theoretical orientation, interpretation may vary widely and do not follow party lines. Jungian analyst Patricia Berry's[11] article outlines 7 divergent Jungian interpretations to a short dream. Contemporary psychoanalytic interpretations may also vary widely, with some focusing on early Freudian instinct-based interpretation of wishes but most focusing on more diverse models of working with dreams, emphasizing issues such as object relations, attachment issues, the regulation of self-esteem, affective and cognitive reorganization,[5] mastery and problem solving,[12] and transference and countertransference.[8]

To show individual differences in interpreting even a common dream theme, let's consider the dream of losing teeth, which is not as common as flying or paralysis, but occurs worldwide. It is often, but not always, characterized by teeth crumbling and falling out. This dream theme can be used to show the limitations of objective and fixed interpretation of symbols and the need to be attentive to multiple levels of metaphoric meaning as well as individual and cultural differences and the timing of interpretations. An interpretation of losing teeth as an objective warning might lead to consideration of concerns about oral health and the booking of an overdue dental examination. A fixed symbolic interpretation, with a classical psychoanalytic perspective, might suggest castration anxiety related to fixation in the early phallic stage of development perhaps set off by current feelings of emotional impotence. A Jungian or cross-cultural interpretation may reference anthropological studies interpreting wearing the teeth of an enemy as a symbol of aggression and dominance. Experiential and existential approaches may recommend reexperiencing the dream and describing the emotional reactions during and after the tooth loss.

Without ruling out the possible relevance of these interpretive strategies, let's consider some additional frequently occurring meanings of tooth loss dreams. In general, dreams of losing teeth occur when there is a narcissistic injury or a blow to a person's self-esteem, a feeling of emotional impotence, or a physical threat, such as an injury or serious or life-threatening illness. In these common scenarios, the crumbling teeth represent emotional or physical impotence. However, when a 6-year-old child loses the first tooth and places it under the pillow and dreams of losing teeth, it is more likely related to excitement about the special attention received from the family. When a newly licensed dentist dreams of losing teeth, the dream may be more about performance fears or financial stresses.

In the author's study of the dreams of the 1991 Oakland Firestorm survivors, Susan, a 44-year-old woman, had to run from her house to escape the wall of flames that swept down the hill, which ultimately burned 3000 homes within a few hours. Six weeks after her home burned to the ground, she had the following dream: "I see the wrong dentist. He makes a mistake and accidentally knocks out my weakest tooth. I am devastated. I weep and then feel grim and angry."[13] During free association, she initially thought of a trip to the dentist to get a cavity filled. That was unpleasant but not traumatic. As she continued to associate to the dream, the dentist reminded her of the insurance adjustor who was trying to seriously reduce the settlement amount from her home insurance company. Exploring the dream made her more aware of the sense of mistreatment, rage, and impotence triggered by the loss of her house and unfair treatment by her insurance company. It also reminded her of other times when she had been treated unfairly and felt she had no remedy or could not fight back, in her family of origin and in her adult life.

Susan Knapp[14] cites the case of a tooth loss dream that symbolized strength rather than powerlessness. The dreamer had consistently worked in occupations that were far below her intellectual potential. She had always acted nonchalant about her jobs, but this facade concealed a terror of failure that kept her from trying out new career possibilities. She had been studying for the Graduate Record Examination to apply to graduate school. She and her husband dwelt on the emotionally catastrophic consequences of her failing to get in. After discussing her husband's attempts to block her career aspirations, she had the following dream. "I dreamed that my teeth were falling out. Then the support system beneath them, which was made of toothpicks, also fell out. But then underneath the old teeth and the new toothpicks was a perfectly good set of new teeth."

Initially, the dreamer seems to be losing her potency, which had been artificially propped up. Dreams exaggerate anxiety, and this part of the dream probably refers to her fear of being powerless or of failing. However, the dream reveals an unusual twist. Rather than experiencing the upsetting, disfiguring loss of a whole set of teeth, she realizes that what she is losing are the false teeth that had covered her real molars. The new set of teeth represented the sense of power that she and her husband had conspired to ignore. Exploring this dream allowed her to appreciate the powerful resources that she had long denied and to move ahead with her career exploration.

It is valuable for psychotherapists to be aware of the meaning of common and universal dreams. However, even common dreams, such as flying, paralysis, or losing teeth, will not always yield to expected interpretations or expert explanations. Every dream must be explored to find the unique meanings that resonate with the life experiences and psychological circumstances of the dreamer.

DREAMS AND LIFE PASSAGES: A DEVELOPMENTAL PERSPECTIVE

Past trauma and early family dynamics may influence dreams, but it is also important to consider the effect of current life transitions. This approach appeals to patients who tend to be receptive to linking dream content to current and pressing life events and passages. It may also provide crucial diagnostic information about how the individual is adapting to transitions in life, such as getting married, becoming a parent, midlife crises, going through the stages of grief, and approaching death.

Studies of dream content have identified developmental changes in dream themes. Children's dreams are shorter with less plot development, and younger children are less likely to be in control and are more often the victim of adversarial forces[4] and are less able to fend for themselves. Most preschooler's dreams feature animal characters, whereas adults tend to have animals in less than 10% of their dreams.[15,16]

Jung observed that extremely vivid and memorable dreams accompany important life crises and transitions. He hypothesized that a weakened ego led to more active unconscious activity and memorable dreams.[17,18] More recently, Rosalind Cartwright's research on the dreams of divorcing women resulted in an intriguing finding that the first REM cycle began much earlier than the usual 90-minute latency between sleep onset and Stage 1 REM. It seems that people undergoing acute crises may have a greater need to dream, which manifests partly through earlier REM onset.[19]

Studies of traumatized combat veterans helped establish the syndrome associated with posttraumatic stress disorder (PTSD), which was first included in the Diagnostic and Statistical Manual of Mental Disorders (DSM) III in 1980 as a unique diagnosis. Intrusive nightmares are one of the cardinal symptoms of PTSD,[20] and recurrent and relatively unchanging nightmares are considered to be one indicator of unresolved trauma associated with PTSD.[4] Jungian analyst Harry Wilmer's yearlong study of the benefits of dream-oriented psychotherapy provided fascinating case studies of Vietnam era veterans who had suffered from chronic PTSD and repetitive posttraumatic nightmares. Wilmer found that twice-weekly therapy sessions featuring dream discussion helped to resolve chronic nightmares and furthered progress in therapy.[21,22]

In contrast to persistent nightmares that arise during the period of reacting and recovering from unexpected trauma, recurrent patterns have been identified in individuals undergoing expectable or anticipated life transitions, such as marriage, pregnancy, grieving, and approaching death. These event-related dreams may be helpful diagnostically and therapeutically and provide a window into developmental and psychological changes associated with these life passages.[4]

Research on expected or anticipated life transitions, such as pregnancy, has identified several common dream themes. These recurring pregnancy dream themes include nurturing or giving birth to furry mammals; dreams of irresponsibility, such as forgetting to care for the baby; infants with impressive verbal and intellectual powers; giving birth to deformed children or animals; dreams of fertility; water imagery; and other metaphors for womb-like environments. Prior studies and the author's clinical and teaching experience show that one of the most frequent pregnancy dreams involves giving birth to animals, often furry mammals. These are likely to be a symbol of the fetus and are emblematic of the parents' emerging relationship with their child and are part of a psychological processing of preparing for the responsibility of parenting. Often, the dream animals are tiny and live in enclosed or watery environments in early pregnancy dreams and are larger mammals (such as dolphins or even walruses) in later pregnancy dreams.[4] The universality of these themes was anecdotally corroborated by the author's discovery in Freud's *The Interpretation of Dreams* of an expectant mother's dream of a brown furry seal emerging from a trap door.[1] It seems that Viennese women expecting children in the later 1890s had similar dream themes to American women a 100 years later.[4]

The content of an expectant father's dreams had some similarities to women's pregnancy dreams, such as watery environments, miraculous male pregnancy and birth dreams, and many sexual dreams. Expectant fathers had dreams suggestive of great excitement about parenting, nurturing significantly more themes of exclusion,

rejection, and abandonment. Many of the sexual dreams had themes of sexual rejection, which may reflect waking experiences of reduced frequency of sex and a more general feeling of rejection often experienced by men. These latter dreams correlate with one of the key developmental tasks faced by expectant fathers, that is, resolving the sense of exclusion that arises as the attention is focused on his wife and he begins to feel more excluded from the developing relationship between mother and child.[4]

Few people are aware of common dreams associated with divorce, pregnancy, grief, or other life transitions, and many people are troubled by these dreams and don't realize they are usually evidence of normal-range anticipatory anxieties. A study of the dreams of women in their mid-pregnancy found that those who had more frequent dreams of threat and hostility ended up having shorter labors and fewer complications.[23] This is similar to Cartwright's finding that divorcing women, whose dreams focused more directly on the emotions related to the separation, showed better adjustment and were less depressed a year later.[19]

Expectable life transitions as well as unexpected crises and traumatic events, are characterized by vivid dreams, and frequently the dream themes are closely linked to the developmental psychological tasks associated with the transition or life crisis. In their dreams, expectant parents are nurturing mammals, worried about the responsibilities of parenting and about mishaps during the birth or about having a baby with problems.

After the death of spouse or close relative, dream content reveals stages of coping with and resolving the grief for months and often years after the loss. These dreams provide diagnostic information that can help clinicians identify blocked or unresolved grief. The dreams also highlight aspects of a life transition that are especially challenging and that can stimulate insights and expedite resolution of conflicts related to grief or other transitions.

COLLABORATIVE EXPLORATION OF DREAMS IN PSYCHOTHERAPY

A participant in the author's study of the Oakland-Berkeley Firestorm of 1991 dreamed of an empty shopping cart after the house she was living in burned down. Her first association was to the homeless people whom she passed by regularly on her way to work. Literally homeless after the fire, her dream also symbolized her emotional and financial depletion. This and other dreams helped her see the depth of her depression, and as a result, she decided to seek psychotherapy.[13]

Patients often bring dreams to therapy because they are upsetting or vivid and because many expect that dream exploration will be an important part of therapy. When a patient brings a dream to therapy, there is a strong desire to receive an answer from an expert who can instantly untangle the riddle of the dream's message. This expectation can lend power and importance to the therapist's response. However, interpretations without an exploration of associations may succeed on occasion but are likely to be premature or not resonate with the dreamer. It also puts pressure on the therapist, who may feel uncomfortable not knowing the answer to the riddle of the dream's meaning. Letting go of the pressure to know the answer is a crucial first step for the therapist.

Donning the expert hat may feel satisfying but can ultimately be disempowering to the dreamer who may take a passive role, expecting to deliver the gift of the dream and in turn receive an answer from an oracle dispensing sage advice. The well-worn adage applies here that feeding a person a fish nourishes for a day but teaching him or her to fish may sustain the person for life. Especially in the initial stages of therapy, teaching and modeling a process of collaborative dream exploration may lead to more productive use of dreams as a source of insight and therapeutic change.

If the patient does not spontaneously bring a dream to therapy, introducing dreams as a possible focus or feature of therapy can be accomplished in various ways. As part of a routine intake when issues about sleep are explored to determine if sleep disorders affect the patient's symptoms or functioning, queries can be made about whether the patient has had nightmares, recent dreams possibly related to their current symptoms, and whether they tend to remember dreams and share them with others. Psychodynamic psychotherapists or those who have had more training in working with dreams may also inquire about recurring or meaningful dreams, posttraumatic nightmares, or childhood dreams. Psychotherapists working with people from differing cultural backgrounds may inquire about relevant cultural or religious beliefs about dreams (see later section for more about cultural dimensions of dreaming). Writing about the use of dreams in brief psychotherapy, Wallace and Parad[24] advocate a strategy of telling the patient in the first session that "dreams are a rich, creative source of material and often furnish answers to current problems, and the progress in therapy can be greatly enhanced by remembering them."

Another issue to consider is whether the therapist should write down the dream during the session, but the therapist may miss the chance to observe the nuances of facial expressions and body language as the patient recounts the dream narrative. On the other hand, for those who do not have outstanding auditory working memory, writing the dream down after the session may lead to omissions and distortions and will be time consuming. If taking notes during a session does not seem unusual to the patient, jotting phrases from the dream may help consolidate the therapist's memory and make it easier to refer back to the dream later in the session and identify patterns in subsequent dreams.

A basic principle of working with dreams is to view the interpretation as a collaborative process involving the therapist and the patient. The process goes through a series of stages that include exploration of effects, memories, ideas, and insights triggered by the dream. This may include a retelling or reexperiencing of parts of the dream, a verbal rescripting or imagining new directions or endings, especially for nightmares and unresolved dreams. It can also involve exploring connections of the dream to current and past memories, conflicts, and relationship and identity issues. After the process of free association comes a brainstorming process, with the patient and psychotherapist forming hypotheses about possible meanings of the dream and testing these hypotheses and connections that allow the dreamer to gain insights that lead to reevaluation or changes in identity, relationships, or other life issues.

A valuable first step in working with dreams is to have the patient repeat the dream. This repeating allows the dreamer and the therapist to savor the imagery and begins to trigger associations as the dreamer spontaneously experiences feelings and ideas while recounting the dreams. It helps the therapist to recall the dream and listen for emotional tone, to watch body language, and to make connections that can lead to suggestions or interpretations as the process continues. There are variations to this technique, including having the dreamer repeat the dream using first person present tense or telling the dream from the perspective of a different character. If patients bring a written copy of the dream, the author first has them narrate the dream without refering to the printed page and then has them read from the page. Omissions and additions usually make for interesting discussion and may highlight areas of conflict.

Freud emphasized the technique of free association for exploring the meaning of dreams and for expert interpretation. Lying on a couch, Freud's patients would simulate a dream state and use the dream narrative as a springboard for making connections to feelings, memories, and ideas. The general principle of free association has stood the test of time as a first stage in dream interpretation. Free association would often lead directly to underlying issues and conflicts, but if taken literally, it quickly diverged away from the dream. For example, a dream of a car losing control may lead to discussion of feelings of losing control emotionally.

Jung's concept of active imagination was a hybrid of free association.[18] It called for loosely focusing on dream symbols and images. In addition to the discussion about feelings of losing control, the dreamer may be directed back to the image to describe other aspects, such as the model of car, the passengers, and the driver. A sputtering Yugo with malfunctioning brakes may have a very different meaning than a speeding Porsche spinning out of control.

Existential and experiential approaches focus on the reexperiencing of all or parts of the dream. This may be easier and more fruitful for some people. For the car crash dream, the dreamer would be directed to imagine and describe the experience of trying to jam on the brakes and the terror of anticipating the crash. This could lead to discussion of past memories of car crashes or other traumatic events, a general sense of loss of control, or other associated memories or feelings metaphorically linked to accidents, crashes, threats, or general stress.

Ernest Hartmann[12] emphasizes the similarities between dreaming and psychotherapy with respect to making connections and resolving emotional conflicts. Dreaming focuses on adaptive challenges facing the individual in the present by metaphorically connecting emotionally charged imagery with related trauma from past conflicts in an instinctive process of resolving current emotional threats. In this sense, dreaming is like a search engine and the dreamer's current emotional challenges are the key words that generate an array of emotionally parallel images in an attempt to assess the nature of the threat to survival and to generate metaphoric solutions. Thus, confronting upsetting emotions and the trend toward integrating disturbing affects and mood stabilization in the dream and in therapy are parallel.

Clinically, this formulation leads to Hartmann's emphasis on the value of focusing on the central image or "the most striking images in the dream."[12] This approach leads "quickly to something emotionally important for the dreamer" and gives the dreamer access to what Hartmann considers the essence of dreaming: "making connections in a safe place." The focus on the most striking images is a user-friendly approach for patients who more often want to talk about the parts of the dream that are most memorable or distressing. Most often, this leads to a discussion and exploration of the most important emotional issues in the dream.

In Clara Hill's[25] cognitive-experiential model of dream work, the first of 3 stages of working with a dream is called the exploration phase, and this phase focuses on encouraging associations. Hill underlines the importance of this stage by recommending the therapist to spend about half the time available to work on the dream. In this stage, Hill likens the therapist to a coach, who guides the exploration process by asking open-ended questions, reflecting feelings, and making tentative restatements to mirror what the client has said. She begins by explaining the procedures and then proceeds to have the dreamer retell the dream, focusing on the emotions, describing and reexperiencing the images in the dream, and then gathering associations and connections to the day residue or waking life triggers. After the exploration, the patient and therapist make an interim summary.

The second part of Hill's model is the insight stage, which is designed to help clients "construct meanings for their dreams."[25] Although still collaborative, the therapist begins to take a more active role, using and encouraging the dreamer to offer tentative explanations such as "the terror of not being able to stop my car reminds me of the mounting pressures at work that I can't seem to get under control." The therapist can offer alternative ideas to stimulate continued brainstorming about possible meanings of the dream. For example, the therapist may suggest a link between the dreamer's mother screaming in the back of the car and performance pressures from his mother that contributed to his being a workaholic who is never satisfied with his successes. If the exploration stage identified the car as similar to an old Mustang he fixed up and drove recklessly during a phase of experimenting with drugs in college, then a discussion of overworking accompanied by a disregard of time for recreation, exercise, and good nutrition may ensue.

Hill continues to caution therapists to restrain their excitement about their insights and watch and listen carefully to which ideas and hypotheses about the dream's meaning seem to resonate or ring true with the dreamer. This serves to keep the discussion on topics that are more relevant to the dreamer and less tinged with theoretical biases of the therapist. In addition, it helps the therapist to understand what the patient can tolerate emotionally and is ready to explore further.

Hill's third and final stage is the action stage designed to explore various strategies "to extend what they have learned during the previous stages to thinking about changes that they may want to make in waking life." Hill suggests using material generated in the exploration and insight stages to identify problematic behaviors and discuss and rehearse alternate strategies for issues such as improving assertiveness, dealing with feelings of isolation, or expressing emotions more often. A final collaborative summary completes the action stage and highlights insights that bear further exploration in future sessions.

The term rescripting[26] describes the creation of alternate endings or creative amplifications of the dream. This concept was popularized in the 1970s by books referencing anthropological studies by Kilton Stewart on the Malaysian Senoi tribe. They supposedly had a utopian society based largely on daily family dream rituals that featured a rehearsal of waking fantasy resolutions of dream conflicts. Subsequent studies revealed that Stewart's writings were largely apocryphal,[27] and although the Senoi probably used dreams, they were dirt poor and far from utopian. Nevertheless, the notion of transforming nightmares using fantasy gained popular acceptance in the 1970s. More recently, imagining fantasy resolutions to nightmares has gained research credibility through the work of Krakow and colleagues,[28] who found that simple techniques involving repeating and rescripting troubling nightmares were effective in treating women who were survivors of violence.

Rescripting can take many forms and can be applied when working with children's dreams. Younger children may not have the patience to free associate extensively but are often responsive to expressing their dreams in creative ways, including drawing and painting, writing stories and poems, and dramatizing parts of their dreams. These approaches can help children feel more confident about their creativity and imaginative powers and give them appealing ways to express and resolve conflicts creatively through the metaphors of the dream. Some therapists encourage adult patients to use visual or expressive arts to discover meaning in dreams that sometimes do not easily yield to rational analysis. Individuals with creative inclinations may continue to explore, rescript, and work with their dreams between sessions, depending on their interest and favorite media. Visual artists paint or draw imagery from their dreams. Expressive artists dance or dramatize aspects of their dreams. Writers use their dreams as a springboard for poetry, stories, or songs.[4]

Psychoanalyst Montague Ullman[29] developed a training technique for psychiatric residents that featured having group members free associate to a dream as if it were their own dream. He eventually turned this method into a format used for experiential dream groups that could be led by professionals or used in a peer group. Ullman required participants in a dream group to preface all associations and interpretations by saying, "if this were my dream," I would feel a certain way or would interpret it this way. Ullman's publications and techniques have been widely adopted in North America and Europe by professional practitioners and participants in the dream sharing groups that Ullman popularized. This technique is effective at generating associations and hypotheses about the dream and showing multiple levels of possible interpretations. This technique also helps the therapists see how much their interpretations can be infused with projections and personal biases that may not be very relevant to the dreamer's issues. Some therapists may use this technique in sessions to send up trial balloons. Again, using the car crash dream, a therapist might say, "if this were my dream, having my mother screaming at me from the back seat would make me feel humiliated and angry." The therapist can use this technique to mentally try out emotional reactions and then ask questions or propose interpretative possibilities and hypotheses for the dreamer to ponder.

In 1987, Fosshage and Loew[5] presented multiple viewpoints on a series of 6 dreams selected from 1 patient's psychotherapy that lasted for more than 4.5 years. With a short family and psychosocial history, the dream series was provided to clinicians from 6 schools of interpretation, with instructions to analyze the dream series and show how to work with the dreams. The approaches included psychoanalytic, Jungian, culturalist, object relations, phenomenological, and gestalt. Many interpretations overlapped, and the use of multiple perspectives to formulate the themes in a dream series created a more nuanced picture of the dream.

Fosshage and Loew's emphasis on using a series of dreams rather than 1 dream is very instructive, as it parallels the psychotherapy experience of working with an evolving set of dreams over time. Because the manifest content of dreams often exaggerates, conceals, or even reverses the polarity of an emotional or relational conflict, working with a series of dreams is an important corrective that helps to adjust and recalibrate hypotheses about the meaning of the dream themes. After reviewing the convergences and divergences in interpretive style among the 6 theorists, Fosshage ultimately settles on his own "revised psychoanalytic approach," emphasizing that dreams are a form of affective-cognitive reorganization. His model posits that dreams use primary processes to maintain, regulate, and reorganize internal images of self and others and cognitive structures of the psyche and "continues the unconscious and conscious waking efforts to resolve intrapsychic conflict."[5]

The value of viewing and comparing multiple approaches to the same dream series is that an eclectic and multidimensional approach produces more nuanced and individualized insights. Clara Hill's cognitive-experiential model capitalizes on an eclectic approach that shows less devotion to 1 school of therapy and is designed to be used clinically and to be studied to determine the effectiveness of using of dreams in psychotherapy with different populations. This is an important direction for the twenty-first century and could lead to improvements in understanding and using dreams in therapy.

UNDERSTANDING CHARACTERS AND RELATIONSHIPS IN DREAMS

Before getting married, expectable anxieties about commitment manifest in common dreams about sexual adventures with former lovers or other appropriate or inappropriate objects of affection. Six weeks before his wedding, Brian reported in therapy, a series of vivid dreams about sexual encounters with old girlfriends. He felt ashamed and guilty and began to doubt that he had made the right decision to go through with the wedding. He had increased symptoms of depression, including disturbed sleep, loss of appetite, and sadness. In one of the dreams, he was amorous with his high-school girlfriend whom he had not seen for more than 15 years. "She wants to make love and tells me she has loved me all these years. I ask her if she is still married. She doesn't answer but I have a feeling she has left her husband."

Although there were no overt conflicts with his fiancé and the wedding planning was going well, Brian was troubled by these dreams and wondered if they were telling him that he was not ready for the commitment of marriage or if he had chosen the wrong partner. Brian had been keeping a dream journal, and as we reviewed some of the other dreams of affairs with old girlfriends and unknown women, most of them involved a sexual encounter followed by rejection. In therapy, Brian had dealt with fears of abandonment that had blocked his ability to commit in prior relationships. As he explored the meanings of these dreams, Brian realized they were not necessarily about desires for sexual variety nor were they literal predictions of rejection or failure if he went through with the marriage. On the threshold of making a lifelong commitment, he was struggling with fears of abandonment.[4]

Other premarital dreams, which I call Bride of Frankenstein dreams, exaggerate personality or appearance defects in the intended spouse. These dreams add to prewedding jitters and are often taken literally as signs of not being ready because of the desire to sow more wild oats or cast doubts on the suitability of the marriage partner they have chosen. As with many anxiety dreams, reassurance can be a valuable and necessary first step to get beyond the panicky feeling that the wedding should be called off. Once the patients hear that prewedding doubts and related nightmares are common, they are willing to consider metaphoric meanings such as how the dreams of affairs may be related to preparing for the commitment by "closing the book" on old relationships or that the temptress in the dream may actually represent attractions for their fiancé. The Bride of Frankenstein dreams may be reversals emphasizing less-desirable attributes of their own personality or exaggerations of minor flaws in the appearance or personality of their intended spouse. For example, Diane was preparing to marry a man who was 5 years younger and dreamed that "My fiancé showed up in a horrible blue suede patchwork jacket and announced that he is feeling trapped. He felt that if he married me, he could not be wild. I think this is odd because before he arrived, I had been flying through the air in a convertible."[30] As Diane explored the dream, she realized that it was less about doubts about her fiancé and more about losing her own wild side as represented by flying around in a sports car and wearing outlandish clothing.

Understanding the meaning of characters in dreams can be complex and requires using multiple lenses to view the dream. It is always tempting to equate the "me" in the dream, as an alter ego, representing the dreamer and the other dream characters, as closely linked to the real relationships the dreamer has to the character. This perspective offers an entree point, has excellent face validity to the dreamer, and may be very productive in generating further associations and insights.

However, the dream characters may be unknown people or famous actors, politicians, or even historical figures or may combine features of known and unknown people. Freud's early descriptions of dream mechanisms, including displacement and condensation, are still worthwhile constructs to understand relationships in dreams. Using displacement, the character, known or unknown, may be a stand-in for a person or type of relationship that is important to the dreamer. A dream argument with a coworker may be a displacement for a conflict with a spouse or sibling. This also fits with Freud's early formulation of the dream as a disguise or camouflage for underlying conflicts.

Condensation is a more flexible and versatile construct for understanding dream characters. Many dream characters condense or combine aspects of someone close to us with other incongruous features. An example is a man in his 40s who reported dreaming about an angry-looking character that looked like his business partner but was shorter and older and dressed in torn and dirty clothes. He was not having any disputes with his partner who was usually well dressed. However, as he explored his associations, it occurred to him that he was worried about his father who was a widower living alone who was becoming increasingly temperamental and hard to manage.

Once we go beyond the notion that dream characters are merely close representations of the people who appear in the dream and current aspects of our relationships with them, there are a few valuable constructs to consider when trying to explore and decode the meaning of dream relationships. The quality of relationships and interactions in dreams may be linked to problematic or changing relationship patterns. For example, in Rosalind Cartwright's[19] research on the dreams of divorcing women, participants in the acute phases of adjusting to marital separation were alone, isolated, and set apart from others. Their dream relationships paralleled the social and emotional isolation and changing sense of identity from being a partner to a single person. Dreamers who are feeling social or psychological isolation or detachment may describe a pattern in their dreams whereby they are a passive observers and not an active participants.

A woman, who had separated from her husband and was considering following through on a plan for divorce, had repeated dreams in which she was single and felt excluded in groups of married couples.[4] One dream was overt and featured her scantily clad in a towel and single at a party of well-dressed married couples. She saw the dream as representing her loss of identity as a married person and current sense of isolation and alienation. A thematically similar but less obvious dream occurred soon after. In that dream, she saw people riding on normal 2-wheeled bikes, but she was attempting to ride a unicycle. Other than scenes from circus, she initially had no associations to the unicycle but was excited in the dream that she was able to actually ride the unicycle. Free association led her to view the 2-wheeled bikes as representing couples and the unicycle as representing her new single status, which was precarious but potentially navigable. The dream helped her feel more confident in her decision to pursue the divorce and survive on her own.

During the process of free association and making connections between dream characters and psychological issues and conflicts, some valuable techniques have been developed, including retelling the dream from the point of view of a different character. Another general technique is to consider the dream characters and even dream settings or objects as aspects of personality. This can be confusing or jarring but often leads to important insights. Chase dreams are common especially in childhood and often involve threatening animals, but adults also dream of being chased by thugs, terrorists, or other evil beings. Description of the terror of being mortally threatened may lead to insights about emotional threats in the past or present and may create a bond between the dreamer and therapist and allow the therapist to witness the dreamer's vulnerability and offer reassurance. However, it is harder to imagine "what part of me is the threatening terrorist filled with rage or vengeance?" The Jungians call this as working with the shadow archetype or the part of the personality we fear and don't own as part of the persona we put forward to others.

Several schools of therapy have encouraged the use of spontaneous verbal or even written dialogs between characters or objects in the dream to unravel the meaning of dream relationships. A variety of dramatic and theatric techniques can generate insights into the meaning of dreams. In one variation, used in gestalt therapy, the dreamer would talk to an empty chair representing the other character or switch chairs to alternate roles. Fritz Perls encouraged a dreamer to have a dialog with a rug that was in a dream. The dreamer soon realized that she felt "stepped on" in various relationships in her life. Other variations suitable for group therapy include having additional people dramatize parts of the dream and then switch roles. The dreamer and the other participants try to get the feel of each dream role and discuss their reactions afterward. Subsequent discussions try to synthesize various reactions, and the dreamer reflects on any insights gained from participating and observing others react to the dream.

DREAMS, DIAGNOSIS, AND PSYCHOPATHOLOGY

Early in his career, Aaron Beck analyzed the manifest content of the dreams of depressed individuals and identified patterns of masochistic themes.[31] Subsequent case studies have revealed general patterns in the dreams of depressed and suicidal people that can be used diagnostically and therapeutically.

Psychoanalyst Robert Litman,[32] a pioneer in the development of the suicide prevention movement in the 1960s, listed a series of dream themes that were commonly encountered in individuals who were acutely suicidal or who eventually killed themselves. These dream themes included death and dead persons; destruction of self, other people, and symbols of other people; and being trapped and struggling unsuccessfully."

When severe depression is present, dreams may reveal themes of struggling and giving up. Litman reported the case of a severely depressed professor, who despite relative success, was harshly self-critical and felt that his life work had been a sham. On the eve of his 40th birthday, which was to feature a party thrown for him by friends, he dreamed that "a large black cube lay in his way as he tried to walk along a path and no matter how hard he tried to move, the cube moved with him. Finally he gave up and merged with the black cube."

One of the most troubling signs of imminent suicidal risk in a severely depressed patient is a sudden remission of symptoms, accompanied by giving away possessions or other evidence of alleviation of depression. This trend may be "signaled by peaceful dreams of taking leave," when the suicide plan has matured. Litman described the dream of a chronically depressed woman who had a history of suicide attempts in reaction to the break-up of a love affair. At age 50 years, she felt that she was no longer attractive, her marriage had little intimacy, and she had not developed a career. After her psychotherapist returned from a vacation, she reported the following dream: "I was walking down the street with my brother and we said goodbye to each other. I turned and walked off the road into a beautiful meadow with flowers and sunshine, peaceful and lovely. He on the other hand, walked on into a dirty, dark, dangerous alley filled with garbage and filth."[32]

Her brother and the therapist were the only people with whom she had a supportive relationship. Entering the nirvana of the meadow and abandoning her brother in the wretched alley were evidence of splitting, which is a defense mechanism common in borderline personality disorders. The patient and the therapist interpreted the dream as evidence of her being acutely suicidal. Because she had multiple prior nonlethal suicide attempts, the therapist did not anticipate the acute nature of her suicidal tendencies. She died of an overdose of sleeping pills the next day.

Dreams may also portend recovery from an episode of depression. Novelist William Styron[33] associates a dream with the beginning of his recovery from an episode of paralyzing depression. This is consistent with research findings that have shown that dreaming is more infrequently remembered or suppressed during severe depression.[34] Increased recall or memorable dreams may herald breakthroughs in resolving severe depression.

When severe or acute psychiatric symptoms are present, dreams may add information that can be a valuable supplement to traditional diagnostic procedures. This is especially relevant when patients report troubling dreams but have difficulty communicating the full nature of their symptoms. When language is a barrier, such as in patients who are receiving therapy in a language other than their mother tongue, dreams may help to understand the patient and lead to important diagnostic hypotheses. For children, who have not reached a level of cognitive development that allows them to fully differentiate dream from reality, being chased or threatened, being abandoned by their parents, or witnessing violence is sometimes more distressing than waking experiences. Because children may have difficulty articulating their distress caused by emotional trauma, anxiety, or confusion, dreams may provide diagnostic information and a vehicle for exploring issues that are hard to express.

Ten-year-old Alexander was referred to the author because of misbehavior at school, including talking back to teachers, and angry outbursts at home. After his parents divorced when he was in preschool, he visited his father on alternate weekends, but his father was increasingly belligerent, constantly bad-mouthing, and even threatening Alexander's mother, calling her a slut and threatening to brandish a weapon if his stepfather picked him up at the end of the weekend visit. He was not enthusiastic about coming to therapy and did not hide his resistance. He initially refused to talk about his visits with his father and became protective toward his father in response to any of my queries that even hinted at any negative appraisal of the father. His mother reported that he began to have repetitive nightmares about being trapped or paralyzed and pushed down on his bed unable to breathe. She encouraged him to talk with me about his suffocation nightmares. He finally agreed, and on the night before the session, he had another nightmare about a time bomb ticking inside of him. He dreamed "I can hear this tick-tock sound, and I can hear the footsteps. I am looking from the view of the guy with the bomb and hearing what he hears. The sounds are getting louder and louder and all of a sudden it explodes."[4]

The time bomb dream was extremely disturbing to Alexander and symbolized the traumatic effect of his father's aggression and his fear that he was becoming explosive like his father. The dream revealed more about his emotional distress than he had been able to communicate and was diagnostically valuable in the therapy. Alexander felt relieved and reassured after sharing the dream and requested that his mother join him in the session. After exploring the dream, he opened up and provided more details about his father's threatening behavior, such as keeping guns in the house and his emotionally abusive behavior. He admitted that he was terrified of his father's temper and often had nightmares after the visits. After a longer discussion, he asked for shorter visits without overnight stays. Because of his revelations, the court required mandated short and supervised visits. This ultimately led to a reduction and eventual cessation of his nightmares and a gradual improvement in his classroom behavior and academic performance.

Dreams can provide valuable diagnostic information and insights in therapy. Like any other assessment tool, dreams should be used along with a full history, emphasizing differential diagnosis and a review of records and consultation with other professionals treating the patient and with any other neurocognitive, medical, or psychological tests.

ETHICAL ISSUES AND GUIDELINES FOR WORKING WITH DREAMS IN PSYCHOTHERAPY

Several ethical concerns about using dreams in psychotherapy have been raised by skeptics and advocates. These concerns warrant careful consideration and suggest strategies that may help avert misguided or unethical use of dreams in therapy. Psychotherapists who have not been trained in working with dreams or have not undergone psychotherapy are most likely to interpret the dream prematurely, to infuse the interpretation with their own projections, or to make strong, pedantic, and seemingly final interpretations without the benefit of free association and collaborative discussion.

Dream interpretation has been criticized as being unscientific and slanted toward reinforcing the theoretical bias of the interpreter. Subsequent dreams are shaped by subtle or not-so subtle theory-based responses of the psychotherapist. This perspective has been amplified by the observation that authors of case studies regularly select dreams that perfectly illustrate the points they want to make. This critique has been addressed, in part, by content analysis studies, which collect dreams in a standardized format and analyze recurring patterns such as gender, cultural, or age differences; reactions to traumatic events; and other issues. Nevertheless, a Jungian who immediately interprets every dark figure as related to the archetype of the shadow or a psychoanalyst who listens selectively for themes of aggression, sex, or oedipal conflicts runs the risk of interpreting dreams in the manner of the nefarious ancient Greek highwayman Procrustes, who would stretch or cut off the legs of his guests for them to fit into the bed.

There are several steps that can be taken to avoid misguided or manipulative interpretations caused by excessive theoretical bias and Procrustean dream interpretations. The first is to be cautious about fixed, literal, and objective interpretations of dream symbols and themes, especially in the absence of thorough exploration of the dreamer's associations. Metaphoric and multidimensional exploration of dreams helps to guard against fixed and reductive interpretations. A second precaution is to make interpretations as tentative hypotheses that get tested in discussion with the dreamer. Even if the therapist is on target, the interpretation may be premature or overwhelming to the patient's defenses. Carl Jung emphasized that an interpretation must "win the assent" of the patient, and his advice has stood the test of time. Check in frequently to make sure the interpretations resonate with the dreamer. A third guideline is to stretch the boundaries of your theoretical biases and become familiar with multiple theories and strategies for dream interpretation and to use them as lenses that allow insights into different dimensions of the dream.

Further ethical concerns were raised during the 1990s, when a trend emerged in a small group of so-called recovered memory psychotherapists to seize on dream content, manifest or latent, that was evenly vaguely suggestive of abuse. By directing the associative process and making reductive interpretations to confirm the abuse based on their dreams, patients were led to falsely conclude that they had been abused, to sue family members, or to take other misguided actions. The American Psychological Association countered this trend by developing ethical guidelines that emphasized caution in assuming that a dream or other evidence of a recovered memory is evidence of abuse without additional corroborating evidence.[35] Nevertheless, renowned memory researcher, Elizabeth Loftus, who was instrumental in debunking the unethical practices of the rogue recovered memory therapists, seized on the use of dreams in psychotherapy as a potentially abusive practice leading to distorted and manipulative interpretations. Although the ethical cautions raised by Mazzoni and Loftus[36] are worthy of consideration, the negative effects they observed in their experimental design were the result of intentional distortions on the part of the experimenters who sought to reinforce a false memory. In addition, the same ethical criticisms they raised could be leveled against any practitioner, regardless of orientation and irrespective of whether they use dreams in therapy.

Ethical concerns about recovered memories and dreams are made more complex because individuals who have suffered severe trauma and abuse that has been objectively confirmed often suffer from posttraumatic nightmares for years to come. Psychiatrist Lenore Terr[37] documented the dreams of the 1975 Chowchilla kidnap victims. After being buried in a school bus by kidnappers demanding ransom, the children dreamed about the trauma for decades afterward. Terr also reported on persistent nightmares in the English survivors of the German rocket assaults on London during World War II. Holocaust survivors, child abuse victims, persecuted political refugees, combat veterans, and other trauma survivors may experience trauma-related nightmares even when they have consciously suppressed or unconsciously repressed the painful memories. Therefore, one must be attentive to posttraumatic themes emerging in dreams but not take dreams with abusive or intrusive interactions as literal evidence of abuse or trauma without corroborating evidence.

Cultural sensitivity is also an important consideration in the ethical use of dreams. We must respect each dreamer's cultural beliefs and experiences if we are to help them understand and benefit from exploring their dreams. When you listen to a dream from someone who is culturally different, be cautious about interpreting until you can learn more about their cultural beliefs about dreams and their symbolism. This will help the dreamer feel more understood and empowered and help the therapist develop a richer understanding of universal themes and cultural differences in the meaning of dreams. The International Association for the Study of Dreams publishes ethical guidelines for working with dreams, with focus on cultural sensitivity and additional emphases on using collaborative and multidimensional perspectives.[38]

Historically, dreams were considered to be divine or diabolical messages from gods or spirits. The incubus and succubus were believed to be spirits that visit or attacked the dreamer during sleep and are examples of cultural beliefs that spirits external to the dreamer are the source of particularly the most distressing dreams. At the beginning of the twentieth century, Freud promulgated and popularized the notion that dreams were intrapsychic phenomena. However, in most cultures, even in the twenty-first century, people respond to their dreams as bearing objective truth, predicting the future or containing literal messages about the status of relationships. Embedded in many cultures are beliefs about what specific dreams symbols mean or even about the nature of dreaming. Many cultures support the idea that dreams featuring communicating with dead relatives are valid experiences. Interpreting such a dream as intrapsychic phenomena may risk alienating the patient and conveying disrespect for their beliefs.

Predictive and precognitive dreams are widely taken literally, and in some cultures, every dream is interpreted as a reversal, that is, the dream is interpreted as the opposite of what the manifest content suggests. Fixed cultural interpretations of symbols may vary widely. For example, some cultures view the color white in dreams as representing birth and purity, whereas other cultures view white as representing death. Because of the varied and sometimes contradictory way in which different cultures interpret dreams, a dream or symbol dictionary may not help, but asking patients about their beliefs and researching cultural differences in dream interpretation may be more fruitful.

Practically, it may be hard to research the dream beliefs of every cultural group you work with. However, for immigrants and minority members in a dominant culture, dreams may give insights into cultural identity and reflect poignant themes of struggles with acculturation and assimilation pressures. A common recurrent dream for immigrants involves a journey back to their country of origin or place of birth.[39] For individuals who are in minority groups in a culture, dreams may contain important references to prejudice and struggles related to assimilation. When a bilingual person reverts to their mother tongue in dreams, it may give clues to their cultural identity and point to important emotional moments in the dream that bear further discussion.

An additional ethical consideration stems from the fact that many professionals have not received training on working with dreams and that most graduate students receive little if any training on theories and techniques of working with dreams in psychotherapy. Most students take the elective course taught by the author toward the end of their graduate training when they have completed the required courses on psychopathology, research, psychological assessment, and so forth. In recent years, very few of my graduate students have had more than 1 class session in which dreams were discussed apart from the physiology of sleep and dreaming. Ethics and licensing guidelines proscribe the use of any technique without graduate or postgraduate training, and therefore it is important for practitioners who work with dreams in psychotherapy to seek some specialized training in working with dreams. This can come from continuing education seminars, supervised work with dreams, reading, or attending workshops. Freud and Jung developed their theories in part by carefully documenting and analyzing their own dream. One of the best training experiences for psychotherapists is to remember their own dreams, keep a dream journal, explore dreams when they undergo psychotherapy, and observe ongoing themes and patterns in their dreams. In addition, psychotherapists who work with dreams will benefit from having case-focused clinical supervision or consultation to familiarize themselves with techniques and theories as well as with ethically and culturally sensitive approaches. Keeping a dream journal, working with their own dreams in psychotherapy, and having a supervised practical training that integrates dream work will enhance skills and minimize the effect of personal and theoretical biases and blind spots that could limit effectiveness in using dreams in therapy.

CLINICAL USE OF DREAMS: OLD WISDOM AND NEW DIRECTIONS

Freud pointed to the therapeutic value of dreams at the beginning of the twentieth century. Dream work for the twenty-first century requires a multidimensional, metaphoric, and individualized approach that respects the culture, beliefs, life experience, and emotional sensitivities of the dreamer. Such an approach calls for caution about imposing theory-based expert interpretations and emphasizes a collaborative and creative process of exploring the feelings and associations triggered by the dream. This is followed by making connections between the dream narrative and the dreamer's emotions, past experiences, relationships, and trauma as well as presenting conflicts and relationships, issues of identity and self-esteem, developmental challenges related to life passages, and possible cultural, existential, and spiritual dimensions.

Advanced training in a particular school of therapy can be crucial, especially if there is an emphasis on the use of dreams. However, whether the practitioner is psychodynamic, Jungian, cognitive, existential, or humanistic by training and orientation, working with dreams calls for an eclectic approach that incorporates techniques and insights from different schools of therapy and focuses on the dreamer's therapeutic needs rather than strict adherence to a theoretical or technical approach. An eclectic and flexible approach using multiple theoretical lenses to understand the dream and diverse techniques to explore the dream may be more effective than relying on a unitary theory or set techniques.

In the twenty-first century, more of the mysteries of sleep and dreams will likely be revealed through research and clinical experience. Perhaps we will eventually be able to holographically record our dreams in 3-dimensional form and revolutionize our understanding of the meaning and function of dreams and use them in therapy in ways we cannot yet imagine. In the meantime, working with dreams adds a dimension to psychotherapy that taps into one of the most fundamental and creative human experiences that is linked to how we adapt to challenges that are crucial to maintaining our identity, sense of meaning, and connections to those we love and to restoring our emotional balance.

REFERENCES

1. Freud S. The interpretation of dreams. New York: Avon; 1965.
2. Domhoff GW. Finding meaning in dreams: a quantitative approach. New York: Plenum Press; 1996.
3. Moffit A, Kramer M, Hoffman R, editors. The functions of dreams. Albany (NY): State University of New York Press; 1993.
4. Siegel A. Dream wisdom: uncovering life's answers in your dreams. Berkeley: Celestial Arts; 2003.
5. Fosshage J, Loew C, editors. Dream interpretation: a comparative study: revised edition. New York: PMA Publishing Corp; 1987. p. 3.
6. Delaney G, editor. New directions in dream interpretation. Albany (NY): State University of New York Press; 1993. p. 5–9.
7. Natterson JM, editor. The dream in clinical practice. New York: Jason Aronson, Inc; 1980. p. xix–xxi.

8. Erikson E. The dream specimen of psychoanalysis. In: Lansky M, editor. Essential Papers on Dreams. New York: New York University Press; 1982. p. 137–79.

9. Breger L. The manifest dream and its latent meanings. In: Natterson J, editor. The dream in clinical practice. New York: Jason Aronson; 1980. p. 9–12.

10. Dement W, Vaughan C. The promise of sleep. New York: Dell; 2000.

11. Berry P. An approach to the dream. Spring: An Annual of Archetypal Psychology and Jungian Thought 1974:58–79.

12. Hartmann E. Dreams and nightmares: the new theory on the origin and meaning of dreams. New York: Plenum; 1998.

13. Siegel A. Dreams of firestorm survivors. In: Barrett D, editor. Trauma and dreams. Cambridge (MA): Harvard University Press; 1996. p. 171.

14. Knapp S. Teaching the clinical use of dreams. In: Ullman M, Limmerman C, editors. The variety of dream experience: expanding our ways of working with dreams. New York: The Continuum Publishing Company; 1987. p. 238–52.

15. Foulkes D. Children's dreams: longitudinal studies. New York: Wiley; 1982.

16. Siegel A, Bulkeley K. Dreamcatching: every parent's guide to exploring and understanding children's dreams and nightmares. New York: Three Rivers; 1998.

17. Jung CG. Dreams. Princeton (NJ): Princeton University Press; 1974.

18. Mattoon MA. Applied dream analysis: a Jungian approach. New York: John Wiley & Sons; 1978.

19. Cartwright R, Lamberg L. Crisis dreaming: using your dreams to solve your problems. New York: HarperCollins; 1992.

20. American Psychiatric Association. DSM-IV-TR. Diagnostic and statistical manual of mental disorders. 4th edition. Arlington (VA): American Psychiatric Association; 2000.

21. Wilmer H. The healing nightmare: war dreams of Vietnam veterans. In: Barrett D, editor. Trauma and dreams. Cambridge (MA): Harvard University Press; 1996. p. 85–99.

22. Wilmer H. How dreams help. Einsiedeln (Switzerland): Daimon Verlag; 1999.

23. Winget C, Kapp F. The relationship of the manifest content of dream to the duration of childbirth in primiparae. Psychosom Med 1972;324(2):313–20.

24. Wallace ME, Parad H. The dream in brief psychotherapy. In: Natterson JM, editor. The dream in clinical practice. New York: Jason Aronson, Inc; 1980. p. 405–26.

25. Hill C, editor. Dream work in therapy: facilitating exploration, insight, and action. Washington, DC: American Psychological Association Press; 2004. p. 41–67.

26. Halliday G. Treating nightmares in children. In: Schaeffer C, editor. Clinical handbook of sleep disorders in children. New York: Jason Aronson; 1995. p. 167.

27. Domhoff G. The mystique of dreams. Berkeley: University of California Press; 1990.

28. Krakow B, Johnston L, Melendrez D, et al. An open-label trial of evidence-based cognitive behavioral therapy. Am J Psychiatry 2001;158:2043–7.

29. Ullman M. Appreciating dreams: a group approach. New York: Cosimo-on-Demand; 2006.

30. Westbrook D. Dreams and first marriage at midlife transitions. Ann Arbor (MI): University Microfilms International; 1989. 51.

31. Beck A, Ward C. Dreams of depressed patients: characteristic themes in manifest content. Arch Gen Psychiatry 1961;5(5):462–7.

32. Litman R. The dream in the suicidal situation. In: Natterson J, editor. The dream in clinical practice. New York: Jason Aronson; 1980. p. 283.

33. Styron W. Darkness visible: a memoir of madness. New York: Vintage; 1992.

34. Armitage R, Rochlen A, Fitch T, et al. Dream recall and major depression: a preliminary report. Dreaming 1995;5(3):189–98.

35. American Psychological Association. Questions and answers about memories of childhood abus. Available at: http://www.apa.org/topics/memories.html. Accessed February 9, 2010.

36. Mazzoni G, Loftus E, Seitz A, et al. Changing beliefs and memories through dream interpretation. Appl Cognit Psychol 1999;13:125–44.

37. Terr L. Too scared to cry: psychic trauma in childhood. New York: Basic Books; 1990.

38. International Association for the Study of Dreams: Ethical guidelines. Avialable at: http://www.asdreams.org/ethics.htm#ethics2. Accessed February 9, 2010.

39. Maduro R. Journey dreams in Latino group psychotherapy. Psychol Psychothe Theor Res Practice 1976;13(2 Sum 1976):148–55.

Index

Note: Page numbers of article titles are in **boldface** type.

sleep.theclinics.com

Moving?

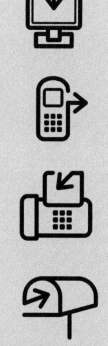

Printed and bound by CPI Group (UK) Ltd, Croydon, CR0 4YY

08/05/2025

01864753-0002